Saskia Calliste

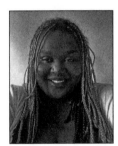

Saskia is assistant editor for Voice Mag UK where she writes about societal issues and reviews fringe theatre, including Edinburgh Fringe in 2019. She freelanced for *The Bookseller* and has had her work published in the 30th-anniversary edition of *The Women Writers' Handbook* (Aurora Metro). She is the author of the blog sincerelysaskia.com, has an MA in Publishing and a BA in Creative Writing & Journalism.

Zainab Raghdo

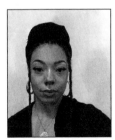

Zainab is a writing assistant and content creator at ContentBud, and the author of the thecoffeebrk.com. She has an MA in Publishing and a BA in English Literature and Classical Civilisation and has freelanced for many years, recently being published in a the new arts journal, *The Bower Monologues*, and the online African Woman's magazine AMAKA.com.

First published in the UK in 2021 by SUPERNOVA BOOKS
67 Grove Avenue, Twickenham, TW1 4HX

Supernova Books is an imprint of Aurora Metro Publications Ltd.
www.aurorametro.com @aurorametro FB/AuroraMetroBooks

Instagram @aurora_metro

Foreword by Stella Dadzie copyright © 2021 Stella Dadzie

Authors' Note by Saskia Calliste & Zainab Raghdo copyright © 2021 Saskia Calliste & Zainab Raghdo

Our History by Zainab Raghdo copyright © 2021 Zainab Raghdo

Her Hair Stories compiled by Cheryl Robson and Saskia Calliste copyright © 2021 Aurora Metro/Supernova Books.

Endnote by Saskia Calliste copyright © 2021 Saskia Calliste

Poems by Kadija Sesay copyright © 2021 Kadija Sesay

Illustrations by Aleea Rae copyright © 2021 @aleearaeart

Editor: Cheryl Robson

Thanks to Christina Webb, Saranki Sriranganathan, Marina Tuffier

Printed in the UK by Short Run Press, Exeter, UK.

ISBNs:
978-1-913641-13-9 (print version)
978-1-913641-14-6 (ebook version)

FSC
www.fsc.org
MIX
Paper from
responsible sources
FSC® C014540

HAIRVOLUTION

Her Hair, Her Story, Our History

by

Saskia Calliste
& Zainab Raghdo

**with a foreword by
Stella Dadzie**

**poems by
Kadija Sesay**

**illustrations by
Aleea Rae**

SUPERNOVA BOOKS

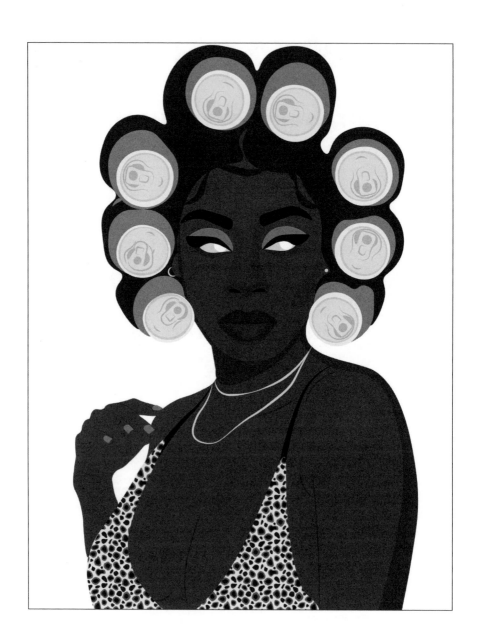

FOREWORD

Stella Dadzie

Have you ever had a really bad hair day that felt like it lasted for most of your life? For many Black women, subjected to a constant barrage of European beauty norms and ideals, this is our reality. At least, it used to be. In recent years, we have witnessed a 'hairvolution' – a quiet revolution in how we see and style our hair – and the trend is increasingly Afrocentric. From complex braids and cornrows to sculptured cuts, dreadlocks, fades and symmetrical Afros, Black women are no longer prepared to deny our hair its natural birthright.

For many of us, the journey to self-love and self-acceptance has been slow and painful. As a people, we have had to contend with centuries of undermining messages, denying us our humanity and mocking every aspect of our appearance – our noses, our lips, our buttocks, our skin and (inevitably) our hair. So different in texture to that of our European detractors, it was an easy target. Untamed hair and savagery were seen as symbiotic. If our tresses weren't combed, curled and compliant, somehow this was seen as evidence of a wild, wanton character, divinely ordained and innately inferior. Viewed through the colonizers' gaze, we were uncivilized, primitive, sub-human beings with the hair to match.

As those of us scattered across the diaspora would soon discover, the word 'beauty' was only ever associated with fair skin and sleek, Europeanized hair. Despite a widespread belief that Black women had lured the hapless white man into a state of lost innocence, officially we were described as the living embodiment of everything Europeans deemed ugly. In a world where a person's race determined their social mobility, many of us did everything possible to disguise our African roots. The kink in our hair, so hard to disguise, was viewed as a mark of shame.

Generations later, we are still grappling with the psychological damage this prolonged assault on our self-esteem has caused us. We are reminded of this fact every time a little Black girl begs to have her beautiful curls straightened because all her schoolmates are white and she longs to look like them. It's not just our children who suffer. You only have to step into a Black hair salon to see the hoops some of us are prepared to jump through in pursuit of this spurious ideal. Harsh chemicals, red-hot tongs, weaves, relaxers, extensions, the list is endless. Shops that sell Black hair products display row upon row of tubs and bottles, all of them promising to tame our unruly locks, many of them eye-wateringly expensive or overtly colourist. It's true, more and more of us are learning the value of natural products – shea butter, coconut oil, products our ancestors used that are tried and tested – but we still have a way to go. By demystifying the experience and shedding light on its long, complex history, books like this will assist us on our continuing hair journey.

Hairvolution takes us back to a time when African women wore their hair proudly, with no fear of ridicule or judgement. It shows how the process of enslavement and mental colonization robbed us of that pride and left us shackled to our own self-hatred. The interviews – my own included – reveal the traumas, influences and moments of revelation that have defined our relationship with our hair. They speak honestly and intimately to an experience many of us will have shared.

For the first time in decades, Black women are reclaiming their bodies. We are strutting our stuff, revelling in our rich diversity. For my generation, the moment of reckoning was symbolized by the Afro – Angela Davis's magnificent halo, so symbolic of Civil Rights and the message of Black self-love and self-reliance. For the Black Lives Matter generation, the icons will be different – the sight of Meghan Markle's mum wearing her locs at the royal wedding, perhaps; or an image of Erikah Badu's wonderfully creative mane spilling from its regal headwrap. Every Black woman who bucks the trend and wears her natural hair with pride is a potential role model, empowering future generations to love and respect their hair.

Of course, whether teachers and employers will see these changes in the same light remains to be seen. We still hear tales of Black children suspended from school because their hairstyle did not 'comply'. Turn up to an interview with your hair in locs, and your chances of getting the job may well have been blown before you even opened your mouth. But attitudes are slowly beginning to move with the times. Perhaps, in the not too distant future, even white folks will recognize that there is room in this world for many different hairstyles, some of which don't aspire to imitate theirs. It's a Hairvolution that is long overdue.

'AIR

Fe-e-e-el this!
Go on!
Fe-e-e-el it!

Soft 'n' wiry all at the same time –
'ow do you people ge' your 'air like tha'?
You people?
Yeah – you culud people.
'Ow am I gonna ge' a brush frew tha'? Tuf' innit?
Bounces back – all springy.
Listen, wha' I'll do for you, love, is,
after I wash i', if it gets any tuffa,
I'll ge' some scissors,
cu' it all orf – might grow back straight
'n' nice'n' long –
then I can brush i' like me gels 'air.
No extra – a-a-a.
Alrigh'?

Gawd Blimey!
Fe-e-e-el this!

– Kadija Sesay

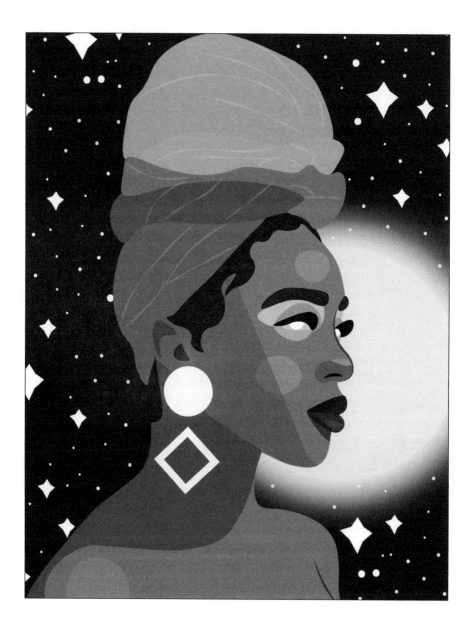

Contents

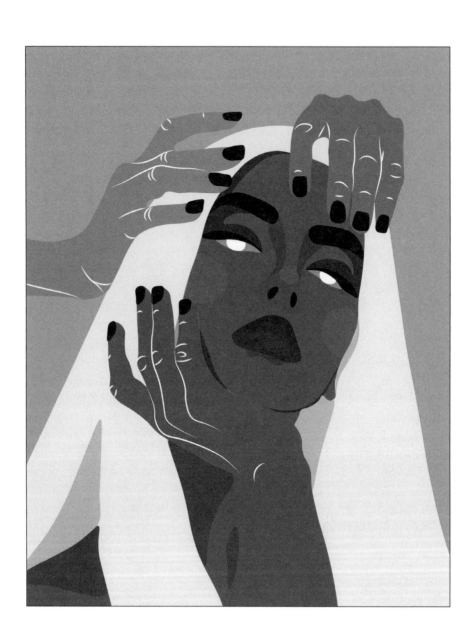

OUR HISTORY

This book is a celebration of our history and culture as Black women. It seeks to affirm the beauty of Black women and, in particular, our natural kinky hair. Western beauty ideals often run counter to African beauty ideals. Where the West has idolized, in women especially, fairer skin and long, smooth, straight or wavy hair, African beauty ideals have traditionally leaned more towards darker skin and kinkier hair that can be fashioned into elaborate communicative styles. Most African hair grows upwards, rather than downwards; it is not "smooth" and "flat"; rather, it coils and springs, and is often braided, twisted, or covered up and adorned with beads, ribbons or ornate fabrics.

Today, especially in our cities, diversity is being recognized as one of the strengths of modern society. Our differences are something to be celebrated, whereas the imposition of one notion of cultural difference over another as being either "superior" or "right" is what has caused the great racial divide that we have seen unravelling before us in the last few years. As a result, Black women living in the West have been judged and assessed against unattainable white beauty ideals for centuries. In the last few years, this way of assessing and valuing women's appearances has created a far-reaching dialogue about our globalized racialized history in an attempt to undo its social consequences.

Although this book has been written in the UK, it aims to cover Black hair and what hair means for Black women internationally; therefore, it is necessary to look at Black hair and hair identity through the lens of African American slavery politics to understand how persisting beliefs and values were formed.

Cultural Identity

Slavery is at the core of every law and social construction that affects the African diaspora.

Its legacy is still with us today due to the sheer scale of the Trans-Atlantic slave trade in which 12.5 million Africans were transported to the New World with only 10.7 million surviving the terrible journey known as the Middle Passage. The number of Africans exported to the United States as slaves during the four centuries in which the Trans-Atlantic Slave Trade flourished is estimated to be around 400,000, while the vast majority of enslaved African were transported to work on the sugar and coffee plantations in the Caribbean islands and South America, with over five million being transported to Brazil mainly by the Portuguese traders.

While much has been written about the treatment of slaves in the diverse colonies to which they were transported, American culture has played a significant part in global consciousness through the influence of Hollywood, American movies and the media. Through this cultural influence, it has affected global reactions to, interactions with and behaviours towards Black people everywhere, but especially in anglophone nations like the UK.

Hair Matters

Hair has traditionally been one of the key ways in which a group of people express themselves. Whether that was to have the hair covered up, worn high, worn in braids around the head or cropped short, hair has never simply been an adornment but has always been influenced by the prevailing cultural and religious attitudes of the time. Hair has changed with the times and the fashions to correspond with developing ideas of beauty, gender identity, morality and medicine, in every culture.

This historical backdrop to the perception of hair in Western European culture shaped ideas about African hair that were to follow. Femininity and individual beauty standards are the first steps to understanding the significance of hair in Africa prior to the arrival of the colonizers from Western Europe and the harmful effect that they had on the continent. Emma Dabiri in her 2019 book *Don't Touch my Hair* explains that in Western African cultures, it was believed that a person's spirit nestled in the hair, as it was the most elevated point on a person's body and therefore closest to the divine. If anyone got a hold of your hair, it was thought – as is still believed by many of African descent today – that they could cause you serious harm. That they could "juju" you, or perform Obeah, cast spells or ensnare your spirit, through the traces of it which remained in the hair, even if it is just a single strand.

This notion of divine hair is a continuous thread that runs throughout pre-colonized African spirituality. One of the most venerated gods in the West African pantheons is Oshun (or Ochún, Oxúm), one of the goddesses of the Yoruba, an ethnic group from West Africa whose descendants in the diaspora can be found in high concentrations in Europe, America and South America. Oshun functions as the mother goddess of the Yoruba pantheon, a primordial deity, one of the manifestations of the Yoruba supreme being and the most important river goddess of the Orisha. She is the goddess of birth, fertility and, most significantly, hair. One of the many symbols of Oshun is the wide-toothed comb or pick, familiar to many of us who have had to use it to get the knots out of our hair, and familiar to our ancestors as a sacred tool through which the goddess Oshun communicated with mortals.

The spiritual significance of hair in pre-colonized West Africa is in no way being exaggerated. Pagan deities and pantheonic deities tell us what is, or was, most important to the people, cultures and societies who worshipped them at any given time. Just as societies such as the ancient Greeks had gods and goddesses associated with the hearth or virginity because these notions were important to their way of life, so too the Yoruba had a goddess of hair, because that is what was most important to them.

Whilst there are few verified images of Oshun left, surviving sculptures and carvings of other African deities as well as wall paintings of Ancient Egyptian gods and goddesses show us that images of the deities almost always coincided with the beauty standards of the cultures and people whom they served. So African deities, like Oshun, looked African, with various types of African hair, body shapes and facial features — and they were considered beautiful because of that. By extension, her worshippers were also deemed to have beautiful, sacred hair and treated it as such.

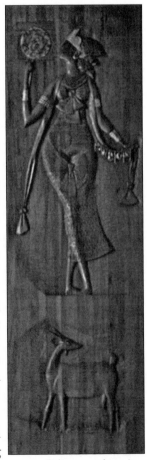

In their pivotal book *Hair Story: Untangling the Roots of Black Hair in America* Ayana D. Byrd and Lori L. Tharps note that, "West African communities admire[d] a fine head of long thick hair on a woman." This "fine head of long hair" was indicative of a "life-force, the multiplying power of profusion". That profusion often translated itself as fertility and showed a woman to be bountiful in her ability to bring forth and raise children. It also suggested that the woman was capable of utilizing the fertility of the earth and the sky, like the goddess, to cultivate the land and bring forth a good harvest to support the lives and livelihoods of those around her.

Hair did more than communicate beauty and fertility. It acted as a means of communicating

Oshun wood carving,
Museum Afro-Brazilian,
Photo: Jurema Oliveira

13

all sorts of messages, both negative, positive and social. It functioned as an "integral part of a complex language system" that helped to structure societies and helped their members to interact with each other without words. But if hair could be a signifier of health and fecundity, it could also be a signifier of ill-health. In Yoruba cultures, if a woman left her hair undone, it was a sign that something was wrong, either that she was bereaved or emotionally unstable. Byrd and Tharps tell us that the Mende tribe of Sierra Leone viewed unkempt, neglected hair as representative of loose morals or insanity; not so different from many of our own reactions today when we see outrageously unkempt hair.

Ethnographer Sylvia Boon noted that the Mende people had a special word for a serious state of unkempt hair, "yivi", showing us just how significant it was for these cultures to be able to determine, immediately, someone's position in society or psychological state from the appearance of their hair.

Hair also functioned as a means of indicating a person's social status within the community: their profession, hierarchy and family name. Byrd and Tharps suggest that a person's surname could be guessed from their hairstyle and that people from the Wolof, Mende, Mandingo, Yoruba, Fulani, Ashanti, Himba and Igbo all had different hairstyles specific to their tribe alone. In Senegal, girls who were not yet of marrying age, or who had not hit puberty, had their head partially shaved to show this. A bereaved woman had to deliberately leave her hair unattended for the specified mourning period. In Yoruba culture, women in polygamous marriages traditionally wore their hair in a "kohin-sorogun" style to show their sister-wife status.

As hair was so vital to the continued prosperity of African communities, the person charged with tending to the hair – the hairdresser – "always held a special place in community life". According to Byrd and Tharps, the hairdresser acted, in part, like a guide, a spiritual medium, and anyone who could master the art of hair and braiding would "assume responsibility for the entire community".

Hairstyling was such a sacred task that, at times, only a family member could be trusted to do it, or you would be assigned a hairdresser from birth to do your hair for the rest of your life. Hairdressing and "hair braiding sessions were a time of shared confidences and laughter; the circle of women who do each other's hair are friends bound together in fellowship". The hair grooming process included, as it still does for many of us, washing, combing, braiding, oiling, twisting and/or decorating the hair with ornaments, including "cloth, beads and shells" and the time spent doing this was considered sacred.

While many African cultures revolved around hair in one respect or another, a large part of that worship, and appreciation, came from the lack of the concept of race. It is always easier to find beauty – or to understand your own beauty to be acceptable – when it's all you know. And for those Africans who had not travelled nor traded with Europeans, there was no concept of a white European race. There was also no concept of a Black race either. In Africa, being Black was the norm, and so was African beauty, including African hair.

The Impact of Colonialism

When Europeans arrived on the African continent in search of trade, they began "Othering" the Africans and recording this process in their letters and writings which were published in books. This meant that their ideas not only survived but were widely distributed. Through this the concept of race was created and the differences between the Europeans and the newly classified Black African race were preserved.

With this new classification came ideas about which race was civilized and which was not. The colonizers sought to justify their exploitation of their fellow human beings by claiming that their set of beliefs and values proved their superiority. They then used their power and influence to impose these ideas on the peoples who were colonized, leading to a loss of appreciation of local cultural traditions by those who were dispossessed. But though race and racial disparity began with the arrival of Europeans, racial hatred did not.

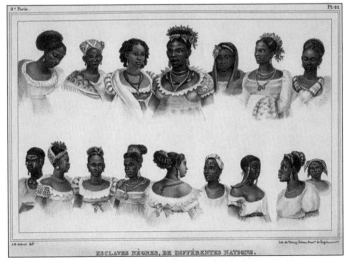

Drawing by JB Debret of enslaved Brazilian women, 1834
Image: NYPL Digital Collections

The Europeans' initial reaction to Africa and African customs was, for the most part, a response of awe.

We know that Europe had a long-standing trading and cultural relationship with North Africans – the Moors – who at the time were considered to be of African origin rather than Arab. These two groups managed to do business fairly amicably for centuries.

In episode one of the BBC documentary *Black and British: A Forgotten History,* British art historian Janina Ramirez and historian David Olusoga refer to Balthazar, one of the three kings said to have attended the birth of Jesus who brought the gift of Frankincense and Myrrh (which were traditionally extracted from Northeast Africa or the Horn of Africa), as being a Black man. The documentary shows viewers a carved, wooden altar piece circa 1530s in Hereford Cathedral, West Midlands, which again depicts one of the three kings as clearly being an African.

His blue robe is adorned with gold. His gold crown is brighter than the crown of the two other paler kings who flank him, and it shines more brightly than any other material in the sculpture. Ramirez explains that his gift in the

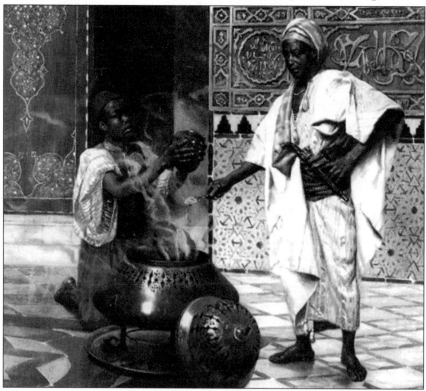

In The Alhambra (a Moorish palace) by Rudolf Ernst. Photo HistoryNmoor

16

shape of a "cornucopia, a horn of plenty," reveals how the medieval European mind saw Africa: as rich, plentiful and beautiful. The figure's position in the image, at the centre with all other activity radiating out from him, suggests that not only was all beauty and bounty extending out of Africa and the African, but to an extent, so did all humanity and Christian religious dignity. Given the subject of the painting, it is unlikely that the artist or the commissioner would have featured such a pivotal character if the African race was thought to be inferior to others at the time.

In the 16th century, as European discovery and colonization of the New World expanded to the North Americas, South Americas and the Caribbean, the Spanish, Dutch, Portuguese, British and French colonialists found themselves in the "unprofitable position of occupying entire islands" with no experience of how to work them.

Having tried to enslave the indigenous people of the New World without much success, the colonizers were discouraged from this by the release of a papal bull – Sublimis Deus – by Pope Paul III in 1537 which prohibited the enslavement of Native Americans. As a result, "realizing the need for an imported labour force, the Europeans reassessed their West African trading partners." To sanction the human trafficking of Africans, some of the European traders revisited a previously passed bull by Pope Nicholas V, namely Dum Diversas which, in 1452, sanctioned the move to "reduce their persons [Saracens and pagans] into perpetual servitude."

This bull gave Catholic Europeans justification from the highest level to make trading arrangements with partners in Africa to capture Africans, who were considered pagans, and commit them to a life of permanent enslavement until, as the name of the bull dictates in Latin, "they are different", a practice which the Protestant traders soon followed.

This idea of "difference" was interpreted to mean that even religious conversion would not absolve the African of the sin of their racial difference. By constructing the concepts of "white", as the purer race versus the Black, impure race, Europeans pitted the two against each other.

Professor John G. Turner in the chapter entitled "The Great White God" from his book *The Mormon Jesus: A Biography*, explains that "a skin of darkness" became a mark of "sin". This deliberately stark language worked within the existing framework of print and literacy in Europe to create the enduring image of the savage, sub-human Black man set against the portrayal of the more enlightened, advanced white man.

Religion and Science Converge

The emphasis on biological differences was taken further by many Christian theorists. According to Craig R. Prentiss in his article "Coloring Jesus: Racial Calculus and the Search for Identity in Twentieth-century America" (2008), European Christians understood "Black" people as pre-adamites, a race of men, or beasts, created before Adam, the true "man". And if man is created in God's image, and the European man is the "real" man, then it follows that the only human that God could possibly accept would be a European, often in English-speaking form. Even the depiction of Jesus was adapted to conform to this notion and, as we know from much of the discussion surrounding the idea of "white Jesus" today, the image of Jesus in churches throughout the world is almost ubiquitously that of a white man rather than a man of Middle Eastern origin. The emphasis on biology and the idea that godliness and purity can only come from "biological lineage" means that those who do not have the right lineage, and who will never be able to attain the correct lineage, would always be sinners; they would always be ungodly, and so, whether they converted or were baptised, they would always be "reduce[d] [to] (…) perpetual servitude".

John G. Turner points out that "the belief that dark skin reflects God's curse was deep-rooted in Western Christianity". The belief was that the sin of Cain, his subsequent banishment and the mark he was cursed with – believed to be the mark of Black skin – was passed on to his ancestors. This was a popular way of explaining the inherent subservient status of the Black race.

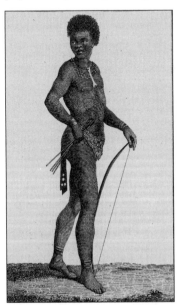

Young "Hottentot" image courtesy of New York Public Library

What's more, by the 1800s, when the benefits of the slave trade were globally acknowledged and the trade was fully established and endorsed, the ideas put forward by Charles Darwin in his books *The Origins of the Species* and *The Descent of Man* inadvertently helped to support the biblical argument for white superiority, whether he intended to do so or not.

Darwin suggested that nature and evolution are based on the "survival of the fittest". And he posited that part of this survival was having lighter skin which made it easier to survive in a stronger, more civilized world — a world constructed by Europeans.

In *The Descent of Man,* Darwin also refers to South Africans, by use of the derogatory term "Hottentot", as "savages" whom he describes as being far closer to our alleged primate ancestors, the apes, than civilized Europeans. He theorized that these savages were examples of the "primaeval man", the missing link, only one step down from the apes, a beast in the evolutionary chain.

What is even more problematic is that he likens the African to an animal, which could be worked and treated in the same way as livestock. All of these negative beliefs and attitudes towards African peoples combined to support the notion of white superiority. This is why white normative beauty standards came into being and why Europeans have been reluctant to deviate from them, long after the justifications for white supremacy fell out of fashion.

Loss of Identity

Edith Snook in her article "Beautiful Hair, Health, and Privilege in Early Modern England" records that European hair received the epithets "Beautiful", "finely textured", "supple", "pliable", with "delicacy" and female characters in prominent European literature, who have the highest moral standing or beauty, are usually described as having fair or golden hair which reflects that disposition.

In literature, these idealized, beautiful, virtuous, elite women – the women with reserves of social capital who are at the centre of romances and love poetry, and are praised for their appearance – have hair notable for its abundance, movement, and slight, natural curl or wave. In all of these works, waving, abundant hair that moves belongs to idealized characters, those possessing virtue, purity, elite status, and bravery – the woman who is an aristocrat, praised for her beauty. Hair has signifying power. It provides rhetorical reinforcement for identities venerated as socially advantaged, with purportedly attractive hair used to insist that its possessor is socially valuable.

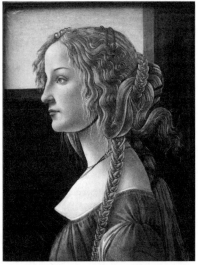

These ideas about hair – what beautiful hair looks like and why the possession of it is so vital – created the white normative beauty standards that Africans could never hope to achieve. In contrast, Afro-textured hair was regularly referred to as "wool or fur", animalistic epithets negating the humanity and morality of the African as prescribed by the religious and scientific theories noted above.

Simonetta Vespuscci by Botticelli, Gemäldegalerie Photo: José L. B. Ribeiro

19

Initially, all of this religious association did little to change the idea of Black beauty in the minds of Black people themselves. The self-deprecation and mental enslavement that would eventually come at the height of slavery did not suddenly take hold just because a person had been captured and put on a ship. To create compliant slaves who would eventually succumb to this way of thinking, Europeans first needed to break Africans. And the best way to break a person is to take away their identity, because separating a person from their home and loved ones alone could not achieve this.

Frank Herrmann, Director of Exhibitions at New York's Museum of African Art, and a specialist in African hairstyles, notes that "a shaved head can be interpreted as taking away someone's identity" and "the shaved head was the first step the Europeans took to erase the slave's culture and alter the relationship between the African and his or her hair".

By taking away this immense cultural and spiritual aspect of African identity, slave traders asserted their dominance over the Africans and in "arriving without their signature hairstyles, Mandingos, Fulanis, Igbos, and Ashantis entered the New World (…) like anonymous chattel".

Once enslaved, they endured brutal and inhuman treatment on the plantations. They had a single meal in a day, with "punishments for insolence, slowing down, or rebellion" which "included whippings with a cat-o-nine-tails, sadistic torture, and amputations of digits and limbs". And given these terrible conditions, it is unsurprising that enslaved Africans had neither the time, resources or the inclination to care for their appearance, least of all their hair and the once "treasured African Combs were [now] nowhere to be found in the new world." The goddess Oshun had been taken from them – no longer held in high regard if she was remembered at all – and their ancient customs were largely forgotten over time.

Slave women also took to covering up the effects that bad diets and a stressful lifestyle had on their hair. The bald patches and matted tresses were covered with fabric scraps and rags which eventually became "ubiquitous to slave culture".

Yet, as the Jamaican saying goes, "turn your hand, make fashion." The enslaved managed to regain the importance of their hair by using the resources at their disposal. Carding combs, which were made for use on sheep fleece, became combs, while the headwrap has been reclaimed and refashioned over the centuries. Many of the headwrap protective styles that we see pop up in the winter today are descended from that tradition of hiding our hair, either when it needs to be protected or when it is undone.

The term 'Sunday best' applied to hair as well as clothes. After a week of having their hair bound up, either to stretch it or hide it, Africans often unveiled their hair on Sundays as part of the Sunday best ritual. A New England traveller in Natchez, Mississippi, described Sunday morning rituals in slave quatres as follows: "In every cabin (...) women arrayed in their gay muslins, are arranging that frizzy hair, in which they take no little pride." Former slave Guz Fester recounts: "In them days all the darky wommens wore their hair in string 'cept when they tended church or a wedding."

In the absence of traditional African hair care products such as shea butter and coconut oil, the hair was maintained by the use of everyday household products. Tracy Owen Pattons in her essay "Hey Girl, Am I More than My Hair?: African American Women and Their Struggles with Beauty, Body Image, and Hair", states that enslaved Africans used "bacon grease and butter" to condition and soften the hair, as well as prepare it for straightening and stretching. "Cornmeal and kerosene were used as scalp cleaners, and coffee became a natural dye for women." All of this shows that despite the atrocious conditions that enslaved Africans faced, one of the few things that kept them going and allowed them to retain their own sense of well-being and self-love was their hair.

Hair Hate

Like the concept of race, hair hate came from the Black slaves' proximity to the white slave-owning families and estate managers and the comparisons that were drawn between the two. Those working in the houses near the slave masters were required to "present a neat and tidy appearance". Unlike field slaves who had to make do with simply what they could get a hold of, "house slaves" could go one step further and often took to wearing wigs, ribbons or styling their hair to look like wigs in emulation of their white masters and to distance themselves from the "nappy-headed" ruffians outside.

European hair, like all other things in a white Western normative culture, became the benchmark by which all other hair was judged. And it was often by their hair that a person was judged — with Afro hair considered as "nappy", "wooly", "unruly", "untidy" and apparently "wild", the reverse of the straight, smooth, neat hair that was considered desirable. So, the need to assimilate arose.

Hair is crucial to the identification of racial heritage, in many ways, more so than skin colour. Dark skin is not specific to the African race, as Polynesians, Indians and Arabs have also been noted to have dark skin, but they are not racially labelled as Black. However, they have still been Othered; they have been dealt with differently by Europeans. As Dabiri rightfully points out, although a large part of the world population is "melanated", "there are few populations beyond those of African descent (…) who have Afro hair" and that is what distinguishes Africans from other darker-skinned people and ethnic groups.

Ingrid Bank, a professor of Ethnic Studies at the University of California, compiled the book *Hair Matters* on the experiences of Black African American women with their hair. In this book, one of her interviewees, Rain, muses that "if she would have had 'measly, short, nappier' hair, she would have been less favoured", supporting the idea that it is hair, more than skin colour, which determines status and racial identity. At the time, status was almost always signified by moral, political and ideological standing, and the more Afrocentric your hair, the more you were assumed to have a low moral, ideological and economic standing.

Inevitably, those who were able to bypass these negative assumptions were Black people with hair closer to the white ideal: Black people with mixed heritage. As a result, the mixed offspring of interracial couplings became the unwitting pawns in this struggle for liberated Black identity. Considered essentially only "half" cursed, having obtained half of their purity from their white parent, having straighter, less curly hair was held up as the ideal, what Africans were to aspire to — as close to being white as the African race could possibly get.

The term "house slave" was widely understood to be a (relatively) better position for a slave to have, as opposed to being a field slave, and being a house slave was usually, though not always, associated with being a mixed-raced or light-skinned, looser curled hair Black person. But Byrd and Tharps point out that, before the solidification of the slave laws in the 1640s to 1670s when the slave trade was still in its infancy and less racially defined, "the scant number of white females, [meant that] some European men sought Native American and Black women for companionship, either by consent or by force". These couplings resulted in children who, because of English Law at the time, were declared to have "inherited the status of their fathers" and could inherit the wealth and land of their slave-owning fathers, and often times owned slaves themselves. Their lighter-skinned and straighter hair spoke volumes of this privilege, or the ability to access this privilege.

By the 1600s, however, the colonies began to reverse this law, and the mixed children of these couplings now inherited the status of their mothers and became "slaves". In the face of this new adversity, "many light complected slaves tried to pass themselves off as free, hoping their European features would be enough to convince bounty hunters that they belonged to the

Enslaved house servants with white children. Sketch from *The Illustrated London News* (1863)

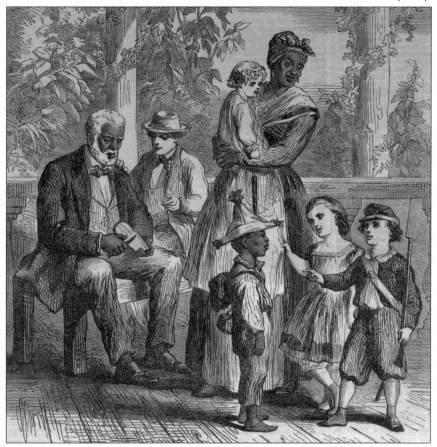

privileged class". But lawmakers, aware of these attempts at passing, made it imperative that no trace of Blackness slipped through the cracks, and the one-drop rule came into effect. It ensured that even the blondest, blue-eyed mulatto would still feel the full force of the white legal system. "The rule of thumb for the one drop rule was that if the hair showed just a little bit of kinkiness, a person would be unable to pass as white". This applied even if a slave had skin as light as many Whites. "Essentially, the hair acted as the true test of Blackness."

And for Blacks whose hair did not show a "bit of kinkiness", it meant a life of, if not passing for free, then at least, "less backbreaking labor (…) access to hand-me-down clothes, better food, education and sometimes even the promise of freedom upon the master's death." As such, there was a constant battle amongst those who could 'pass' to make sure that they maintained and showcased their "good hair". White people were also aware of the significance of long kink-free hair. It was said that "female slaves with long, loosely curled hair" would often as punishment have their "lustrous mane of hair" shaved off by the "jealous mistress".

What's more, runaway slaves were always described as having "bushy hair". And for advertisements of runaway slaves with loosely curled hair, readers were warned not to be fooled by the "long black curld [sic] hair", implying that the long head of loose curls generally denoted an innocence and morality of character that this particular runaway slave had forfeited with their rebellion.

And this idea of "good hair", a term many of us have heard growing-up, began here. "Good hair", the finer, looser curls, typically associated with, though not exclusive to, mixed Blacks, is ladened with all of the cultural and historical implications that came as a result of this slavery environment. It implies breeding, wealth, freedom, education, good manners, good morals, good lifestyle and all of the relatively enviable trappings of existing in slaveholding countries as someone whose physical appearance bore a closer resemblance to that of the dominant white elite. By contrast "bad hair", as many of us have been taught throughout our lives, however unwittingly, is "African hair in its purest form".

In the years leading up to the abolition of slavery, the Free Blacks with extremely light skin and straight hair became known as the "'mulatto elite'" as they still enjoyed a sense of freedom and riches unknown by Blacks with darker skin.

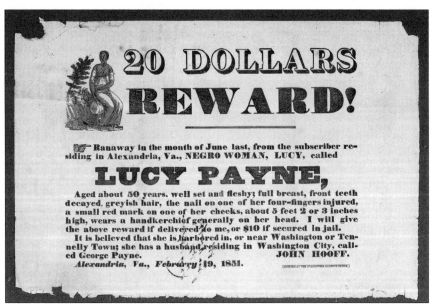

Princess Olive of Haiti

And the maintenance of the physical attributes needed to achieve this status was something that mulattos, quadroons, hexagoons and octoroons fought to preserve well after the abolition of slavery. "They were adept at segregating themselves in tight-knit communities" where they married only other Blacks with similar light colouring and straight hair; they lived in neighbourhoods with people who looked like them and only associated both professionally and socially with people of a similar skin-tone.

Light Privilege

Historical Black colleges, set up for the betterment of the whole Black race (such as Howard University in 1867, Hampton in 1868 and Spellman in 1881), had the unspoken admission requirement of having a "skin tone or hair texture that showcased a Caucasian ancestor". They only catered to those with "the right background and look" as an estimated "80 per cent of students were light-skinned and of mixed heritage". Fraternities and sororities at these universities also only catered to those with light skin and "good" hair, and many of their student parties chose attendees based on the "ruler test" where only "partygoers whose hair was as straight as a ruler would be admitted".

The same went for places of worship where morality and good character were measured by proximity to physical whiteness. Entry into the church service was only admitted if the churchgoer passed the paper bag test, a test that measured skin tone by comparing it to a brown paper bag – if you were any darker than the paper bag then you would be refused entry. Another test was the comb test. According to both Byrd and Dabiri, the comb test, a prelude of the Texturism we see today, measured the level of kink in the hair. If the comb could pass through the worshipper's hair without getting snagged on a kink, entry was given; if not, entry was denied.

And whilst all of this is most certainly unfortunate, it is important to remember that in a society where Black is at the very bottom, any means by which to climb a rank or two higher would have been taken. Many Black people were still working on plantations after abolition, despite the change of laws, for lack of a place to go. The introduction of new vagrancy laws also prevented mobility and can be seen as a precursor to the school to prison pipeline system currently in the US today. It shouldn't, therefore, be surprising that those who could avoid this, by displaying their loose curl patterns and lighter skin, did everything in their power to do so.

Around this time, more Black people – women in particular – were beginning to tap into the emerging market of skin bleaching creams and hair straighteners to distance themselves from their African heritage and gain more class mobility. Companies arose to meet the needs of the new Black consumers who now had a little more money in their pockets.

Black Entrepreneurs

At the turn of the 20th century this "new negro era" gave birth to an entirely new concept: the Black entrepreneur, someone who could see the potential and willingness of the new Black consumer to spend their money to get ahead in the new world. The Black entrepreneur knew their customers and knew that the one place Black people would turn to time and time again, to attempt to better their situations in life, was hair. Two of the most famous figures to come into this space were Madam C.J. Walker and her mentor Annie Malone.

Annie Minerva Turnbo Malone, who had a background in chemistry, began thinking about ways to aid the growth of the hair of women who looked like her and who commonly suffered from baldness and hair breakage due to their difficult lifestyles and inabilities to access a proper diet and hygiene. Dissatisfied with the range and availability of hair care products and styles for Black women, Malone sought to find a way for women like her to improve their standing in the world by making their hair more "manageable" and improving its quality. In the 1900s Malone claimed that she would revolutionize Black hair growth with her "miracle hair grower" which she started selling door-to -door in Illinois, marketing it as a "miracle cure" under her company Poro.

One of her sales girls was a young woman called Sarah Breedlove, later Sarah C.J. Walker. Breedlove was born on a cotton plantation farm in 1867 and came to Malone after suffering severe hair loss as a physical response to a mental breakdown caused by her first divorce and her long, hard labouring hours as a washerwoman. Breedlove believed, like many other Black women of her generation, that if she could improve her hair, she could improve her life. So, Breedlove started buying Malone's Wonderful Hair Grower to improve her hair and her life. She became a Poro saleswoman to Malone's clients, selling the Wonderful Hair Grower, presumably by telling them her story of failure

Right Annie Malone
c. 1910

Below Sarah Breedlove/
C.J. Walker
c. 1914

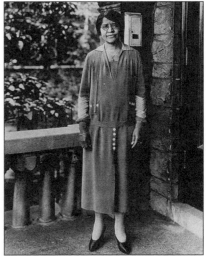

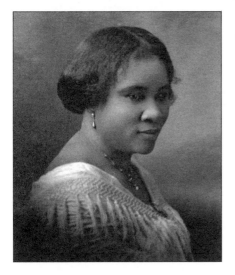

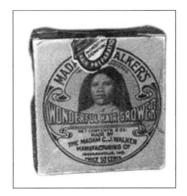

Right above C. J. Walker's
Wonderful Hair Grower in the
permanent collection of The
Children's Museum of
Indianapolis
Right
C.J. Walker driving with friends
c. 1911

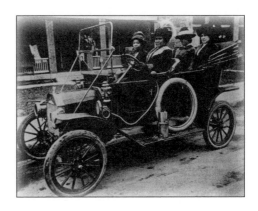

and success through hair. But Breedlove's success with Malone's hair grower is as much a story about representation as it is about Black entrepreneurship.

Malone managed to achieve her success because she was speaking to a generation of women who had never had anyone take interest in their beauty standards before, and they had never had anyone who looked like them telling them that they could achieve beauty. Breedlove's success came from sharing her story of hard work, hair loss and depression – a story that many women at the time would have been familiar with. Indeed, the benefits of the hair grower were clearly visible on Breedlove, a woman who looked, felt and experienced life like them. She had stronger hair, greater confidence and a job, which convinced her customers that they could experience these results for themselves.

Breedlove, by this time Walker, taking the name of her third husband, went on to create her own hair care empire to rival Malone's. And it was because of this idea of representation, and relatability, that Walker was able to do this.

Walker took Malone's hair grower and went on to create her own line of Walker System hair products. It started with the shampoo-press-and-curl: a "method of hair straightening that was to become the foundation of the Black beautician industry". Into this system, Walker gradually included Hair Grower, a pomade called Glossine, Vegetable Shampoo, Tetter Salves and Temple Grower. For her salesgirls, Walker provided a training course kit which included a hot comb, the tool Walker was credited with introducing to the US market. All of these products were designed to help with the specific hair needs of the "New Negro Woman".

These events were dramatized by Netflix in their 2020 drama series *Self-Made* which centres around the growth of the Walker hair company and the rivalry between Walker and her former mentor Annie Malone. The Netflix show makes it very clear that Annie Malone, refashioned as Addie Monroe, is a "light bright", "high yellow woman" profiting off the insecurities of other Black women. In the show, Addie Monroe, played by Carmen Ejogo, uses her own straight, long, mixed hair as the archetype, and uses only fair-skinned, straight-haired women for her advertising and door-to-door sales, forcing all Black women who come to her to aspire to look like her,

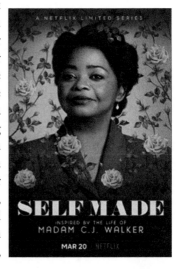

while knowing that most of the time this is unattainable. As a result, Monroe manages to consistently profit from her clients' adherence to an unattainable beauty standard and she revels in being the poster girl for that beauty standard. In contrast, Walker, played by Octavia Spencer, is a darker-skinned, Afro-hair textured Black woman out to better the lot of all Black women everywhere by showing them their own African beauty, rather than demonstrating to them how far from the ideal they are.

Contrary to what *Self-Made* would have us believe, the reality was not so black and white. Malone was not a lighter-skinned Black woman out solely to profit from her clients' insecurities, nor did she set herself up as the epitome of beauty. And Walker was not a benevolent manufacturer out solely to better the community. She was a businesswoman and, as such, was out to make a profit in the same way as Malone by focusing on the insecurities of her clientele.

Walker, again using her relatability to her clients, played on the common preoccupations that come with having non-standardized hair types and used that knowledge to draw her customers in. A 1920s Walker advertisement poster featured a beautiful woman, a flapper, standing at a mirror admiring herself, as do many adverts aimed at women, even today. The advert was depicted as an engraving, so the colouring of the woman is unclear, but it is fair to assume that the woman in the image is lighter-skinned. The figure's hair is quaffed in a 1920s flapper style, a common style for women of the time, and does not celebrate Afro hair. Coupled with the bold assertive title, "You, too, may be a fascinating beauty", there is a clear implication that by purchasing Walker's products you can come to look like the woman in the advert.

There has been a lot of criticism concerning these messages that Walker and Malone provided, claiming that they were "telling Black women to straighten their hair". On the one hand, the relaxer now allowed Black women to gain the "neatness" that white beauty standards demanded of them, but it also meant that the emphasis had now shifted from trying to love their hair in its natural state to, once again, venerating and emulating the white ideal. And many people were very aware of the double-edged nature of Black hair care. The right hair could easily be obtained, even if it was to the detriment of your real hair, and was obtained by a whole generation of women to help them live their lives as best they could. But gaining that kind of hair left many women disillusioned with their heritage. They could not see the beauty of that heritage because they had been taught to hate their hair and were given a quick fix solution on how to eradicate it.

Because of this double bind, hair became the focal point and, in a way, the byword for Black identity more generally in the years after the abolition of slavery, right up until the start of the Civil Rights Movement. It became a means of sympathizing with Black women, telling them not to be a slave to white standards, but it also became a way of ridiculing them for the internalization of these standards.

Black Activism

Popular activists like Malcolm X *(below)* and Marcus Garvey were very vocal about this fact. Marcus Garvey, a Jamaican pro-African activist and leader of the United Negro Improvement Association, in a speech asked his listeners not to "remove the kinks from your hair" but "from your brain". Many Black newspapers, such as the *Crusade*, and Black ministers provided that same message to their readers and congregations, admonishing them for engaging in "unnatural and ungodly habits".

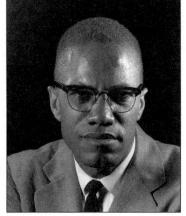

These same sentiments were echoed by Malcolm X whose views are all the more believable and poignant. Though male, X had experienced all three states of the Black hair journey that many Black women transition between in their lifetime: natural, relaxed/permed and back to natural. Although relaxing was more popular amongst men at that time than it is now, it was still a predominantly female practice and few men were writing about their experiences with hair. Because of this, X's testimony can be used to understand a little bit about the psyche of the Black people who relaxed their hair and then gave up the practice.

Malcolm X said:

"The first really big step towards self-degradation: when I endured all of that pain, literally burning my flesh to have it look like a white man's hair. I have joined the multitude of Negro men and women in America who are [so] brainwashed into believing that the Black people are 'inferior' ... that they will even violate and mutilate their God-created bodies to try to look 'pretty' by white standards ... we hated our African characteristics. We hated our hair. We hated the shape of our nose, and the shape of our lips, the colour of our skin ... This is how [Whites] imprisoned us. Not just bringing us over here and making us slaves. But the image that you created of our motherland and the image that you created of our people on that continent was a trap, was a prison, was a chain, was the worst form of slavery that has ever been invented…."

Malcolm X maintained through his speeches and his writings that Blacks who had been "'colonised mentally' would not be able to break the chains of racism until they learned to love their appearance".

This was a sentiment that people such as W.E.B. Du Bois, who criticized Walker, began to take. There would be no real emancipation until Black people loved their hair. And it's an idea that we see repeated today in many inspirational posts on social media and self-love books. But what rhetoric like this fails to acknowledge is that adopting attitudes which champion natural hair and African styles can only follow physical comfort and security. Many of those who ridiculed the relaxing of Black hair and advocated Black beauty were in an economic or political position to do so. People like Du Bois, who already had naturally wavy hair, looser curls and lighter skin, had little to lose by speaking out against relaxers. But those whom they criticized – the shop workers, labourers, teachers and receptionists – did not have the luxury of this mental emancipation. Their primary concern was assimilation and surviving in a society which discriminated heavily against them.

The Windrush Generation

In Britain, the 1950s and 1960s looked very different for those in the African diaspora. Though Black people had existed in the UK for centuries, the roles they could play were limited. They tended to be either the offspring of wealthy British landowners and Caribbean slaves or they were visiting sailors, merchants, Moorish diplomats or African royalty. During the long period of slavery, many were brought from the Caribbean to work as domestic servants in the grand houses built by the plantation owners in Britain. Some ran away and became free men and women, making a living as best they could.

The city of Liverpool, being the largest slave-trading port in the world, was no stranger to Africans on her shores. The exploitation of natural resources and free Black labour in British colonies created enormous wealth back in the motherland which fuelled the Industrial Revolution and the expansion of the British Empire. But after the two world wars, the nation, now in a state of disarray, needed more citizens to rebuild the war-torn country and, as a result, called upon its overseas colonial subjects to help.

In 1948, the *Empire Windrush* made the first of many voyages across the sea to British shores. On this ship were Caribbean immigrants, many of whom were from the Island of Jamaica, and many of whom were, predominantly, of African descent. Some of them were simply answering the call of the motherland, others were ex-servicemen looking to stay in the country they had fought for, and there were those seeking a better life. The British population at the time was generally unaccustomed to the concept of Black people and did not welcome these new arrivals. But the Caribbeans who arrived on the *Empire Windrush* had been educated to respect the motherland; they were hyper-aware of Britain and their connection to it.

Jamaican society in the early to mid-20th century, though very different to that of the US, retained the same social hierarchy of the fairer-skinned people on top and the darker-skinned at the bottom that British slavery had left behind. Stuart Hall in his book *Familiar Stranger* explains that in Jamaica in the 1930s and 1940s, the term "Black" was "taboo, unsayable, especially for the middle classes in Jamaica".

While the term "Black" may not have been used, Hall asserts that "the overwhelming majority of Black Jamaicans clearly understood their racialized inferiorization, from humiliating encounters of daily life to the way that society had been organized by its racial hierarchies".

Independent schools like SP Ardenne in Kingston, Jamaica, which my mother attended, as one of the few darker-skinned women amongst many mixed children even by the 70s, tended to take only those from elite families and these tended to be the mixed or fairer-skinned, loose curl-haired offspring of landowners or foreign diplomats.

The stately homes of governors were often worked by those of the darker-skinned, lower or slightly lower classes. For example, Andrea Levy's *Small Island* illustrates this through the character of Miss Jewel, Hortense's grandmother. The character of Hortense herself, though Black, is taken in by her lighter-skinned, wealthier uncle because her "light skin (…) the colour of warm honey" set her apart from the "bitter chocolate" skinned lower classes like Gilbert and Alberta. Hortense cannot even bring herself to call Alberta her "mother" because of the psychological effects of colonization.

But as Britain was across the sea, it had little need nor inclination to enforce these rigid hierarchies post-slavery, and the more loosely structured colourist society in Jamaica enabled for more freedom of movement between colour and texture boundaries, with everyone being united under the concept of being Jamaican and being British.

For many Jamaicans, like my grandfather, the son of a slave born into the new slavery-free British colony, and for some of my aunts and uncles, there was no concept of "us" and "them". It was simply "we". Jamaicans were treated, in Jamaica at least, as a part of the British Isles. Those who came on the *Empire Windrush*, like those who came from other islands such as Trinidad and St Lucia, travelled on British passports and thought of themselves as British subjects, a title which they held with pride.

In the BBC documentary *Fighting for King and Empire: Britain's Caribbean Heroes*, presented by historian David Olusoga, Caribbean ex-servicemen who fought for Great Britain in World War II and then came back on the *Empire Windrush* to settle in England were interviewed about their experiences. Many of the interviewees note that "in school throughout Britain's Caribbean Colonies, West Indian children were raised with a sense of loyalty to king and Empire".

Ex-servicemen Jake Jacobs and Allan Wilmot who both came to live in England on the *Empire Windrush* recall that in the 40s and 50s, there had been common rumours going about in England that where they came from, presumably Africa, as the general British population didn't know any better, people had "tails" and "in coming to Europe they got the tail cut off, but the stump was still there". Allan Wilmot recalls that "when we came here it's like we dropped out of the sky. Nobody knew anything about us."

Journalist Gary Younge in the BBC documentary *Black is the New Black* also explained that his mother, a *Windrush* passenger, was "shocked that people didn't know Shakespeare and the Magna Carta, because in Jamaica that was what we were raised on". West Indian children were required to know "what each [British] province supplied, where the jobs were". They grew up with this idea of "Hengland" as a country with rolling green hills and the streets of London being paved with gold. At schools in Jamaica, students were taught everything good that there was to know about the "Mother country Hengland" and the curriculum up until the late 1970s was almost exclusively British, teaching all English literature from Shakespeare to Dickens and Tennyson,

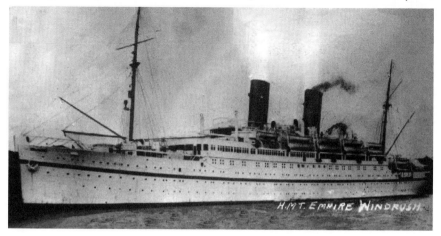

and everything about the ideal British way of life, reinforcing the idea in the Caribbean, and Jamaica in particular, that they were British citizens.

Likewise, in Andrea Levy's *Small Island,* Hortense's grandmother, though of the darker lower classes and continuously mocked for it, is well-versed in the ways of England, as we can see when Hortense teaches Miss Jewel Wordsworth's famous 'Daffodils' poem which she "had learned to recite at school".

But when they arrived on British shores, free, eager and able to work and make a life for themselves in Britain, public sentiment towards these new arrivals quickly soured. For Caribbeans of African descent arriving in England for the first time, the discriminatory behaviour they experienced was a shock.

The Black characters in *Small Island* are frequently referred to as "swine", "monkeys", "golliwogs", "sambos" and "niggermen", all reflective of the attitude that the British exhibited towards Black people in England at the time.

It was demonstrated not only by landlords who would not let rooms to Black tenants, but in the companies who would not hire Black people, or, if they did, who would mistreat them. This was a time when signs were frequently put up in public establishments such as guest houses and pubs which read "no Blacks, no Irish, no dogs", demonstrating the degree of hostility they faced.

The newly created NHS service, which was being propped up by Black nurses, declined to support them against racism from within, and patients routinely refused care from Black nurses. This was the experience of my aunt

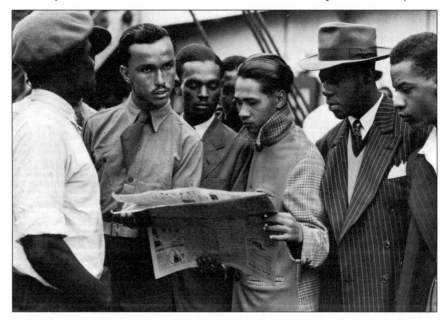

Caribbean passengers waiting to disembark from the ship, 1948, Tilbury Docks, Essex

when she came to England to work for the NHS. The Afro-Caribbean staff and labourers who sustained the transport system were regularly subjected to verbal abuse. And with events such as the white riots in Notting Hill in 1958 and the stabbing of Kelso Cochrane in 1959, the underlying racism within British society reasserted itself.

All of the racially motivated crimes, coupled with the harsh winters and poor living conditions, created a hostile environment that eventually resulted in homesickness in Caribbean immigrants – and more than a little bit of regret. There used to be a saying in Jamaica when my mother was growing up, that anyone who went to England went mad. But many of those who did feel depressed, homesick or regretful did not have the means to, or had too much pride, to return home.

Because of this hostility, pockets of strong Black communities in areas like Birmingham, and Tottenham, Lewisham and Brixton in London, popped up to allow for people to stick together and provide for each other. Ex-serviceman Sam King recalls that when many of the West Indians arrived in England off the Windrush with nowhere to go, they were taken to "Clapham deep shelter and the nearest labour exchange was Coldharbour Lane, Brixton".

As such, Brixton and the surrounding boroughs became anchors for people of the African diaspora arriving in south-east England. In these areas, Black people banded together and bought properties, just as Sam King did in the 1950s when he became one of the first Black people to buy a house in Camberwell. And after providing each other with food, shelter and jobs, hair care was the next service needed for Africans and Afro-Caribbeans to provide for each other.

Black Hair Salons Flourish

In the *Moving Here* series on the Web Archive, *Good Grooming and Reconstruction,* images of popular hairstyles of the time such as the 'Eton crop' are accompanied by notes. In these notes, the Archives' creator Carol Tulloch explains that women like "Beryl Gittens, a trained hairdresser" who had "planned her journey to Britain from Guyana", took her pressing comb with her, which was for the best. When she arrived, she found virtually nowhere to get her hair done and "there was a severe lack of public hairdressing facilities for Black women and men during this period." Mrs. Gittens, who trained as a hairdresser in Guyana from 1947 to 1950, remembers the difficulties this situation caused: "there was nowhere you could have gone into to have your hair done in a white salon ... they could not even comb our hair. And they were so scared of it, they said 'we can't do your hair', and often they never tried, and so I had people who used to come, you see the girls now cutting their hair off, that's just what they resorted to, just cut.'"

Tulloch explains that to address these issues "and answer the pressing need, the Trinidadian pianist, Winifred Atwell established a salon in Brixton in the late 1950s to train English women how to style Black hair". Unlike food and clothes that could be traded for English food and fashions, hair was the one area in which this was not possible and extra care had to be taken to ensure that this precious piece of Black identity was not destroyed by inexperience and tendency to simply burn the hair or "cut" it off. And as the Black community in Brixton rapidly grew, so too did expressions of Black identity, hair being the most notable one. And so numerous hair shops, hairdressers and barbershops shot up around Black populated areas.

Tulloch also reports that "Mrs Gittens opened the first Black hairdressers on Streatham High Street, in 1962" an area with a high concentration of Black people and Beryl's Hairdressing Salon "was the first Black hair salon in London".

As it was in ancient times when the African hairdressers were sacred for being able to help you communicate with the divine through your hair, hair salons today are necessary spaces where Black people can be themselves, both verbally and physically. They are spaces where, as Nadine White writes in her article for the *Huffington Post*, "Black people who are far too often ostracized

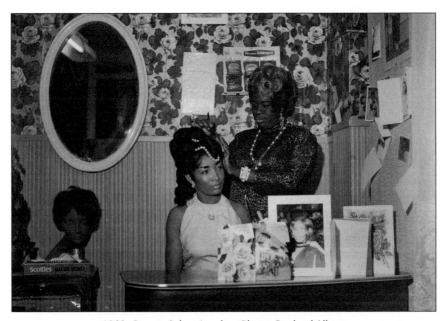

1960s Beauty Salon, London. Photo: Raphael Albert

can either laugh or cry, or both, and their lived experiences resonate with those around them in a way that isn't often guaranteed across wider society".

In these spaces, the person doing your hair understands you. It may only be through an understanding of what to do with your kinks and curls, but in a society that makes you feel outcast, that is enough. Many of us have travelled to more Black populated areas for our haircare needs, and still do, no matter the distance, because the sheer density of the Black population in areas like Brixton in South London means that the paraphernalia of Black homeliness and identity are strongest.

Love Your 'Fro

In the 1960s and 1970s, Black hair took on a whole new meaning. It was a time of cultural revolution and radical thought, a time when men and women of all races in Western Europe and North America were re-evaluating their roles in society and what was expected of them. With this era came the hippy movement, counter-cultural dialogue, and a desire to get back to nature and reject capitalist social structures. All hair was showcased during this time. White people wore their hair long and unstyled to communicate that they were in support of the natural movement, in support of a person being one's self and in support of free love. Black people did the same. In the US, there was a rise in Black consciousness and Black power, which trickled over into the neighbouring Caribbean islands like Jamaica where they were now beginning to think of themselves as Black societies, following the "cultural revolutions of the 1960s and 1970s". This rise in Blackness in the US, the Caribbean Islands and the UK resulted in a style that eventually became symbolic of revolution, rebellion, Black unity and activism: the Afro.

The Afro, however, was more symbolic than natural. Dabiri pointed out in her interview with Matt Elton on the BBC History Extra podcast in 2019, that in West Africa, before the interference of Europeans, Afro-textured hair was rarely left out, uncovered or unbraided. This is not the optimal condition in which Black hair can thrive, as the coils can become dry which can increase breakage. So, the Afro hairstyle is not 'natural'. It does not harken back to a pre-colonized Africa but instead was formulated specifically to showcase the Black hair strands in all of their glory. It was a socio-political statement.

The ideal Afro was large and round; it took up eye space and acted as a call to the Black hair and the Black identity movements associated with it, such as the Black Panthers. It said: we, like our hair, are here to stay, we only grow larger, more powerful and more prominent with time. Look at us, for we will not be erased in the same way that our hair refuses to be erased, by the ever-popular ideas of "neatness" and propriety which white society has imposed on African hair. The hair became our rallying cry.

The style was then adopted by Black activist groups such as the Black Panthers both in the US and the UK, and members of both parties were frequently photographed demonstrating with full Afros.

Byrd tells us that it was between 1964 and 1966 that "Negros" became "Black people". Assanta Shukur, the mother of Tupac Shukur and former member of the Black Panthers, points out that prior to the movement, the term "Black" held the same connotations as the N-word, not because it was actually a bad word but because of how ugly and degrading being Black was thought to be. She recounts: "Black made any insult worse. In fact, when I was growing up being called 'Black' period, was a grounds for fighting. We would talk about each other's ugly, big lips. And flat noses. We would call each other 'pickaninnies' and 'nappy haired.'"

Byrd adds, "To be told that your hair was nappy was akin to having someone talk about your mama."

To suddenly be proud of being "Black" was a revolutionary idea. And this understanding of being Black, unified under one term rather than separated by words such as Negro was revolutionary in itself and could only be achieved through Afro hair, the one thing that all Africans across the world have in common.

The "Negros", the subjugated, enslaved African people and their descendants in the Americas and the Caribbean, were now part of the united Black whole, sharing an identity with anyone whose hair could Afro, creating cross-cultural, cross-border affiliation.

"Black people wore their hair and said something about their politics. Hair came to symbolize either a continued move towards integration (…) or a growing cry for Black power and nationalism. Many African Americans began to use their hair as a way to show a visible connection to their African ancestors and Blacks throughout the diaspora. It was an era in which hair took a prime spot – right next to placards, amendments and marches — in defining a Black identity for the world at large."

As the Afro had become political, Black hair now stood for a return to Africa and Black power; thus, it unified Africans in the diaspora. Africans in the Caribbean, Europe, on the African continent and in the USA began identifying with the message of the Afro simultaneously.

The phrase "Black is beautiful" was first coined in the 60s, when the first 'natural hair movement' began in the UK. There are many popular stories of people falling or being shot at and being saved by their Afro, which fed into the Afro propaganda machine.

One of the most visible women to sport an Afro in the 60s and 70s was Angela Y. Davis, whose outspoken left-wing speeches attracted much public hostility. The backlash against her challenging of the status quo led to her being charged for murder, and serving a prison term, before eventually being exonerated of the crime. Public perceptions can change, though, and Davis was included in *Time* magazine's list of "100 Most Influential People of 2020".

However, recent caricatures of the Obamas which depict them as having Afros, despite neither of them sporting this do, indicate that the Afro with its appearance of unimpeded, free growing, gravity defying, Black hair continues to be regarded as a political statement.

In a world before Covid-19, where going to the office from 9am to 5pm was vital to many people's everyday existence, the concept of 'neatness' and 'professionalism' held firm. By the 80s and 90s the Afro lost much of its political meaning, and receded to being just a hairstyle, and one of many that Black women were able to adopt as a means of self-expression.

People like Grace Jones, Lil Kim, Lauryn Hill and Erykah Badu became known for their heavily Afrocentric hairstyles. Women were inspired to choose which hairstyles they wanted and to be judged not as being rich, poor, morally good or bad, but as themselves.

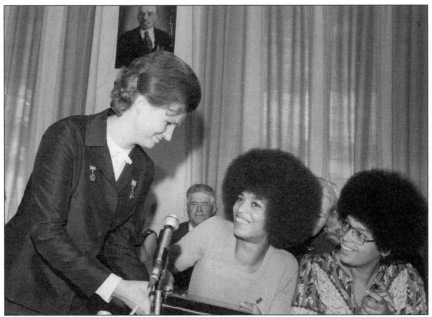

Valentina Tereshkova handing a memento to Angela Davis, and Kendra Alexander *(right)* 1972

Byrd and Tharps claim that hair in the 80s was now labelled as "fun", and the 80s were "determined to liberate follicles from any political and sociological weight". Black hair was, once again, an adornment. Even white people began flirting with the idea of cornrows and braids because they were now nothing more than "fun styles", while professionally, Black hair continued to be judged as improper. Black people, at least in the "professional" sector, were forced to conform to white standardized styles, and the rhetoric around good hair and bad hair continued.

In her book *Hood Feminism,* Mikki Kendall describes how "respectability politics" affect the ways that today's society views Black women. Whilst natural hair and hairstyles were being made popular by the aforementioned artists, they were still heavily stereotyped as styles for creatives or low-income women – people who did not, and could not, exist in the corporate and professional worlds because "respectability", the driving component in all of these environments, was the domain of white men and the occasional white woman.

Because of this, relaxer sales in the latter half of the 20th century and the early part of the 21st boomed, as did the advertising around relaxer. In his article "As Soft as Straight Gets: African American Women and Mainstream Beauty", Ernest M. Mayes looks at various adverts which attempt to sell relaxers to Black women. In all of these adverts the same message is communicated: you can't live a full life without straight hair. But the tactics of many of the adverts which popped up around the later 20th century were far more gendered. Where Walker ads and the rhetoric of previous decades had focused on the need to pull one's self out of poverty, later advertising chose to try and tap into more particular and stereotypical female desires: finding a mate and raising children, which, again, according to the big corporations, could only be achieved through straight hair.

As with any form of advertising, what's being sold is never the product – it's the idea that the buyer can somehow gain some sort of happiness by purchasing this product. As with Walker ads, many of the women featured in adverts for "good hair" are not really selling relaxer, not on its own; rather they are selling the subconscious idea that Eurocentricity is the currency for social and professional fulfilment. One fundamental way in which this is done is by telling consumers a potential life partner would prefer a Black woman who looks white.

As time went on and integration started, the Black man, when not being hounded by the law, was portrayed as the noble savage who could be saved by being with a white woman. For Black men, this idea of the 'noble savage' led to dark-skin becoming fetishized as more masculine, more primal and more sexually gratifying – a thing of awe for the white woman. While this fetishization is problematic, for the most part, it works in the Black man's favour.

For Black women, on the other hand, those same primal characteristics attributed to her male counterparts are what make her, in the eyes of white society, less feminine and more manly, butch and aggressive.

For instance, the Christmas 2020 TV advert by UK supermarket Sainsbury's caused much uproar. One of the main concerns white viewers had with the advert was not that there was a Black family on television celebrating Christmas – because that had been depicted before – but that it was an entire Black family: a Black man and a Black woman together with their children, enjoying family life.

The tweets of several Instagram celebrities, which explicitly likened women with dark skin to animals and sanctioned violence against them, have resurfaced in recent years. This demonstrates the internalization of ideas that have been passed down for centuries: that dark-skinned, African women with Afrocentric features and hair are more masculine, less attractive and more unnatural in a way that light-skinned women with Eurocentric features could never be.

Whilst 21st century feminist criticism seeks, rightfully so, to reject any justification of a woman altering her image for the sake of the male gaze, or the gratification of anyone other than the self, most of us are programmed on some level with the primal need to attract a mate. So, if social attitudes promote the idea that the only way to attract a mate is to alter your appearance in order to look like the ultimate mate – a white woman with sleek straight hair – then that is exactly what women will do.

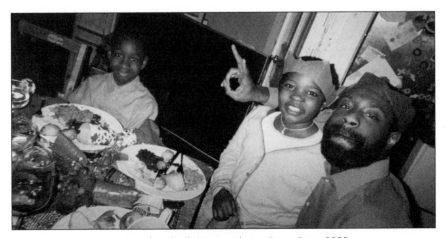

Sainsbury's Christmas advert, *Gravy Song*, 2020

It was Franz Fanon in his revelatory book *Black Skin White Masks* who first articulated the idea that the Black male's pursuit of the white woman was both a means of validating the Black man's freedom (by being able to now take from the white man as the white man had once taken from him) and a means of showing that the Black man had come up in the world. He no longer had to settle for a Black woman who had always been portrayed to him and the world as the lowest of the low. H. Ikard writes in "Rejecting Goldilocks: The Crisis of Normative White Beauty for Black Girls", from his book *Blinded by the Whites: Why Race Still Matters in 21st-Century America,* that in an age when social mobility for Blacks was still limited, Black men, like Black women, were being conditioned to see whiteness as the normative standard by which to excel. And, if they were unable to get a white woman to fulfil that standard, they would settle for the next best thing: lighter-skinned women, whom they had been "conditioned" to see as "one step down on the social ladder, below white women (who were largely off-limits to Black men, legally and otherwise) (...) Black men actively pursued them [light-skinned women] as lovers and wives". It is this social conditioning that plays into advertising aimed at Black women who seek to attract Black mates who prefer, but often can't have, white women.

Spike Lee's advertisement agency knew this when they created the 1998 billboard advert for The Bone Strait Relaxer System. Byrd explains that "The ad showed a woman with long straight hair her head slightly arched back. The caption read, 'My hair. Your man. His fingers. Your drama.'" Byrd explains that the billboard caused "outrage for many (of all races) who felt that the campaign lacked cultural sensitivity and portrayed Black women as sexually licentious home wreckers". However, it was African American women alone who saw the malicious link between long, straight hair, that could have fingers run through it, and the ability to catch a mate. And, in this case, it was to catch a mate from another woman, who according to the advert, did not have the Eurocentric tresses of the relaxed haired woman, and therefore, by definition, was more Black, more unattractive, and less capable and worthy of keeping a mate.

And once a mate is found, if children should follow, Black women were still expected to look to white women, the model for all things correctly feminine, on how to be a good mother. In 1996, a Pretty N Silky relaxer appeared in the May issue of Essence magazine. Many people who grew up over the last 20 years will be familiar with the sight of relaxer packaging, particularly from companies like Dark and Lovely and PCJ, as they tend to grace an entire section in beauty supply stores and beauty salons. The ritual of having to go and buy one of these brightly coloured, brightly packaged boxes before a treatment is one that most of us are familiar with because for many of us it was a must. On the PCJ relaxer box, these ideas are expressed in just a few short sentences.

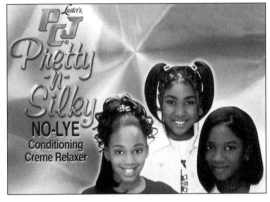

The heading of the ad reads: "Mommy gives us PCJ Pretty N Silky because she loves us!" Below that is the sub-text: "That's right I don't take chances when I relax their hair. I only use PCJ Pretty N Silky children's no-lye relaxer. Its improved conditioning formula has less harsh chemicals than most other relaxers so it's virtually irritation-free and PCJ's NutrientSheen conditioner keeps their hair soft and silky. That's why I trust only PCJ'S Pretty N Silky. Mothers trust PCJ Pretty N Silky."

In the advert, three smiling figures are pictured, similar to the image above. In the centre is a Black woman, not dark-skinned, flanked by what appears to be her two daughters, also not dark-skinned, all with relaxed hair. The figures seem happy, loving and content. The name Pretty N Silky holds all sorts of connotations, namely that one can only be "pretty" if one has "silky" hair while the mother's comment implies that any mother who doesn't relax her children's hair doesn't love them.

This is, of course, an advertising tool. But to dismiss it as simply the company attempting to make a profit would be foolish. Like Walker ads, this advert taps into the unspoken fears of many Black women – of being perceived as masculine, unfeminine and uncaring, and producing offspring who could never survive the world before them. This idea is repeated on the boxes of many other relaxers such as Dark and Lovely's Beautiful Beginning and Soft N Straight No-lye relaxer, and the Africa's Pride 'Dream Kids' relaxer. The message is that if a mother deliberately denies her daughters access to that Eurocentricity, not only was she unfeminine, but she was also a bad mother.

Dabiri asks people to dismiss the idea that all Black hair straightening is a case of "the grass-is-always-greener" vanity and draws attention to the fact that a US federal court made it legal in 2016 to fire a female employee for "unprofessional" hairstyles. For "unprofessional" read Black.

In an age where people are always on the lookout for overt racism, calling our hair unprofessional is the easiest and seemingly unassuming way to channel covert systemic racism and ensure the continued attempted erasure of the Black race.

In many schools and workplaces both in the USA and the UK, it is still legal to exclude students and employees for wearing natural hairstyles. In 2019, California became the first state in the USA to ban discrimination against a person's natural hair in schools or in the workplace. Dabiri points out other instances of this kind of discrimination which is still happening in UK schools in her article "Black Pupils are Being Wrongly Excluded Over their Hair. I'm Trying to End This Discrimination".

In 2019, five-year-old Josiah Sharpe was banned from the playground at breaktimes and eventually sent home from school due to his 'extreme' haircut (a basic fade). He was eventually allowed to return when his hair grew back to what the school deemed an appropriate length. In 2018, Chikayzea Flanders – a pupil at Fulham Boys school – was told he had to cut off his dreadlocks or leave the school. The school only backed down after his mother launched a campaign supported by the Equality and Human Rights Commission. Most recently, Ruby Williams came out of a three-year legal battle with her school in Hackney, where she had been repeatedly sent home because her natural Afro hair was deemed to be against uniform policy.

The message being sent in these instances is very clear: that the natural hair that grows out of the head of a Black person is still as unacceptable, undesirable and as unrefined as it was in the 1600s. If you Google both "professional" and "unprofessional" hair, the images you get are astonishing, with professional hair mostly being made up of white, Caucasian straight hair, versus the unprofessional hair which, for the most part, is simply African hair or hair done up in traditional African styles, braids, dreadlocks, Bantu knots and cornrows.

This idea has been so internalized by Africans in the diaspora that even when we are in environments where straight hair is not necessary, we continue to cling to these mental shackles. Ingrid Banks reports that one of her interviewees remarked: "Although she did not have to straighten her hair to get her job or keep it, she still believed that Black women have to have straight hair to get a front-office job."

Even when a Black woman is excelling at everything in life, her hair remains the focal point of discussion in a way that white feminism would never allow to happen for a white woman.

When they were born, Blue Ivy, the daughter of Beyoncé and Jay Z, and North West, the daughter of Kanye West and Kim Kardashian, were pitted against each other in the media because, despite being the child of two of the most successful musicians and entrepreneurs in the world, certain commentators criticized Blue Ivy for being "ugly". Bloggers like Sandra Rose ignored all of the generational wealth and childhood innocence that Blue Ivy had and instead chose to focus on her personal belief that it was a "shame that Beyoncé brought her daughter out in public with her nappy hair looking like buckwheat". Conversely, North has routinely been praised as the most beautiful baby on the planet because of her loosely curled hair.

Women Against Women

American Olympic gymnast Gabrielle Douglas, after winning two gold medals in the 2012 Olympics, had her enormous achievements and hard work overshadowed by comments that her hair needed to be "tamed", that people "hated the way her hair looks" and that she had "bad weave". And most of these comments come from other Black women, proving exactly how deeply ingrained the psychological conditioning of anti-Blackness is. Popular Black comedies and shows like *Norbit, My Wife and Kids, A Different World, Fresh Prince of Bel-Air* and Disney's *The Proud Family*, though harmless for the most part, routinely cast a darker, either wig-wearing, brightly dyed or kinky-haired woman as the overbearing, loud, obnoxious, devious, masculine, 'ratchet' or antagonistic character in opposition to the woman with light-skinned, naturally loosely curled hair who is the soft, gentle, beautiful, kind and caring female lead.

The trend continues into wider media, such as the classic P. Diddy video for "Need A Girl Part 2" which does not showcase any dark-skinned women as being desirable, nor a single woman with kinky hair. Other videos from artists like Usher, Trey Songz and Tyga have all followed this pattern of showcasing only light-skinned or white women, always with straight hair in their music videos. As Ikard points out, "From hip hop videos and movies to fashion magazines and even video games, the message that darker-skinned women are the most unattractive women on the planet is hard to ignore."

And, arguably, simply accepting this belief is a short-term solution. It allows a Black person to get a job, launch their book, movie or music video, win awards or hit number one in the charts. It serves us as adults, economically or socially, to conform to the standardized ideals of beauty for the physical well-being of ourselves and the next generation.

Talking about such issues has long been a taboo in Black communities all over the world. In part because as a race, the African has endured so much that she does not wish to acknowledge that there is a divide within the ranks as well. However, if not challenged, children, females in particular, will continue to grow up in highly prejudiced, hypocritical, and occasionally hostile environments. They will continue to exhibit the same traits of low self-esteem, shame at being Black and having African hair that their forbears experienced before them, regardless of whether they are physically privileged or not.

Relax – Don't Do It

The revival of the natural hair movement in around 2014 tried to put a stop to the need for chemical relaxers and straighteners. Many women put down the relaxer, and in the age of high-tech social media, there was increased worldwide discussion of these issues amongst Black people globally. More and more natural hair bloggers and events popped up on Instagram and YouTube, all aiming to discuss Afro-textured hair and what it really means to thrive as a "natural". People started sharing their hair stories online and doing "the big chop", cutting off the chemically processed or damaged part of their hair to go natural or go bald. And the message of this movement was that all-natural hair, the hair that grows in its natural form out of the Black woman's scalp, is beautiful as it is, and there is no need for chemical interference.

However, "good hair" is a concept so deeply ingrained in the Black consciousness, merely calling for disposal of chemical interference does not put an end to long-held attitudes, nor does it claim that kinky, tight-curled hair is beautiful. And that has been the overarching issue with all-natural hair movements, to date. The problem is not with the message, but the manipulation of it. In celebrating "natural" hair, without attempting to tear old constructs down, what the natural hair movement actually celebrates is naturally "loose curls". Whilst calling for all hair to now be natural, it does not reassure people that kinky, bushy hair is valued as being "good hair" too.

Arguably, one of the most damaging concepts created by the post-woke 21st century natural hair movement was the concept of Texturism. Texturism is the identification of the curl pattern of a person's hair, ranging from 1A, being bone straight, Caucasian hair, to 4C, being true West African hair. The point of this identification, born out of the 20th century curl test, was for people to be able to identify what kind of hair texture they had in order to select the best products for their hair and tailor their hair care regime to suit their hair type specifically. And, in many ways, it can be useful. Understanding how 3B hair differs from 4C can help you ensure that you are using the right oils, shampoos and creams for your hair and not just using any general "Black hair" product.

Nevertheless, despite the good intentions of Texturism, the whole point of its existence is to measure proximity to whiteness, whether that measurement is for a good purpose or not. And where there is a measure for proximity to whiteness, in a society that still values white beauty standards, there will always be those willing to exploit that fact for personal gain. Companies such as Shea Moisture, one of the pioneering companies of the new natural hair movement, came under a lot of scrutiny in 2017 for marketing their products to all "natural" Afro textures but creating products which seemed to benefit only a certain type of natural hair. They also came under a lot of fire for almost exclusively using models with 2B–3B hair to advertise their products in a 2017 ad campaign while calling for all of their buyers to love their natural hair. Shea Moisture's primary target audience – Black women – was represented in this advert by a single, racially ambiguous, though presumably Black, woman in the top right-hand corner of the advert. The remaining three women being told to "love their natural hair" were all white women.

And whilst 2B–3B hair is indeed natural, these are not the types of curl patterns that need assurance of their beauty. They have been adored both within and outside of the Black community for centuries, and this group does not represent the majority of Black women. It is women with 3C–4C hair types who need assurance and representation – to be told that their natural hair is beautiful – because these are the hair types that have historically been looked down on.

Mikki Kendall explains that "Texturism (the valuing of certain textures of hair above others) in the natural hair community is rampant. In many ways, it is an outgrowth of (…) colorism." Companies and influencers who employ the Texturism argument as a means of celebrating the natural hair movement are causing irreparable damage to those Black women who want to be self-confident in their natural hair, as modern society is telling them to be, but who don't have the "right" type of natural hair.

What is all the more telling, is that many of the major hair brands that do promote natural hair, and endorse the Texturism argument, such as Cantu and Pak's cosmetics, are not Black owned. These companies, owned by white and occasionally Asian men, create products which claim to be for all-natural Afro textured hairs, but many Black women have noticed that they actually provide no benefit to hair that is above 3B. This seems to suggest that the people behind these companies, while creating products which claim to be for "natural" Afro hair are only really catering to the Afro hair that they deem acceptable – kink-free Afro hair.

It seems that a Black woman cannot wear a wig, or else she is told she does not love her natural hair. She cannot relax her hair because it is damaging both mentally and physically. She cannot leave it out or else she will get told she looks a mess, and she most certainly is not allowed to love her natural hair because she is not represented in the media often enough, or positively enough, to feel that her hair embodies the correct type of femininity and beauty that makes her worthy of existing in Western European society. But she also cannot do her hair in an African style because it is 'unprofessional'. And though the media tells her that they want natural hair and that natural hair is beautiful, they are not referring to her natural hair; not the real African hair that grows out of the head of a purely West African woman.

Although the Black Lives Matter movement has brought attention to systemic racism in many areas of society, African hair remains to this day a thing of ridicule in every century and every society that exists under the watchful gaze of white supremacy, whether it is overt, covert or institutionalized.

The Way Ahead

Tracey Owens Patton notes that when TV was first introduced to Fiji, a society of women who were traditionally curvy, shorter in stature and high in self-esteem, they suddenly began exhibiting low self-esteem, eating disorders, such as anorexia and bulimia, and a lack of confidence in their own beauty. For many, this change seemed inexplicable. But Patton notes that this shift coincided decisively with Fijian women's new exposure to TV and the images of idealized Anglo-American women. Suddenly, a society of women who had never experienced any form of beauty but their own were faced with the awful realization that they, despite being the majority and ideal beauty standard in Fiji, were, in fact, the minority beauty standard in the countries that apparently mattered more. This example illustrates one irrefutable truth: tell a girl that she is beautiful, show her beautiful women around her who look like her and she will believe that she is beautiful. But remove all positive images of women who look like her and replace them with unattainable standards of beauty, as well as negative representations of the women who do look like her, and she will inevitably internalize these beliefs and be convinced that she is ugly.

As children, most of us have a shared hair journey up until a certain point. Most of us have a story of relaxing, scalp burns, traction alopecia, hair breakage and the final decision not to take it anymore. Kendall relates that "because of how I was raised, I used to be one of those Black women who thought natural hair looked a mess" – which, at some point, has crossed the minds of all of us. And hair, and our ideas about hair, live on in our collective consciousness. Good hair and bad hair are ideas we have grown up around, and though the terms are seldom used now, they are ideas which all of us innately understand because we have been raised by both our families and society to understand them. The details of our experiences may change but the general consensus is the same. We've all thought at one point in our lives or another: you are not beautiful if you are too dark, and nappy hair is ugly.

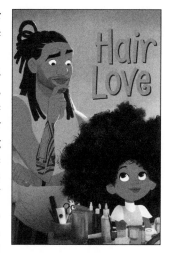

But in recent years there has been some extra push by prominent figures such as Emma Dabiri, Issa Rae, Ava Duvernay and Lena Waithe for more deconstruction of this harmful narrative. Their continued push for movies and books featuring dark-skinned, kinkier haired women – like Jodie Turner-Smith in *Queen and Slim*, Lupita N'Yong'o in Jordan Peel's *US* and Issa Rae in her TV series *Insecure* – all aim to portray dark-skinned, Afro-haired Black women in positive, normal, leading roles. And the effects of this cannot be understated. Like the effects of TV on Fijian women, positive representations of the self are key to the idea of self-love.

When the 2019 award-winning film *Hair Love* came out, many of the comments by viewers expressed the idea that they, the adults, wished they had been able to see it when they were young and that they were glad that their children would be able to see it now. *Hair Love* tapped into a need that is sometimes downplayed within the Black community: to love one's own natural hair in all of its forms. The film's success at the Oscars indicates that it not only engaged with its audience, but that there also has been a shift within the media and Black culture towards positive representations of Black hair.

The educational element of the film cannot be ignored. In representing a Black man doing his daughter's Afro hair, the film also attempts to undo a narrative that Black history and existence are always an offshoot of slavery and can instead be – as they often are – stories of love, community and creativity. Teaching the next generation that they are the inheritors of more than just shackles and chains, of loss and pain, will build a pride that extends to all of the things that embody that Blackness – specifically our hair. Moreover, one of the first places to start doing this is in our use of language. As simple as it sounds, doing away with terms like "good hair" and "bad hair" can make a huge difference in the way that younger Black people interact with their hair. Taking terms like "bushy", "dry", "picky", and replacing them with more positive words such as "springy", "thirsty" and "cute" can, in the long term, do away with the ideas so many of us have had throughout our childhood – that Afro hair is a burden to be dealt with, rather than a blessing to be nurtured.

Reclaiming our own hair care is another major step on this journey to self-love. By creating our own products, we can ensure that all of us are represented. Brands like Afrocenchix, Taliah Waajid and Mielle, all of which have popped up in the last few years, are all Black and female-owned, and are all aiming to cater to all-natural hair types.

As Stuart Hall artfully puts it, "Contrary to common sense understanding the transformations of self-identity are not just a personal matter. Historical shifts out there provide the social conditions of existence for a personal and psychic change in here." And that is in part the purpose of this book: to change and understand the language of hurt that many of us have experienced and to be a part of the shift out there which will enable all of us to have a personal and psychic shift in here.

Our hair is not just hair. It's our history, our affirmation and, for many of us, particularly now, it's a living testimony of our own resilience in a society that would erase Black people, like it would erase the kinks in our hair and the melanin in our skin.

It's not just hair. It's our heritage, and it's time for our Hairvolution!

Bibliography

Ayana D. Byrd, Lori L. Tharps. *Hair Story: Untangling the Roots of Black Hair in America*. New York: St Martin's Griffin, 2014.

Banks, Ingrid. *Hair Matters: Beauty, Power and Black Women's Consciousness*. New York: New York University Press, 2000.

Black is the New Black. Produced by BBC, 2016.

Dabiri, Emma. "Black Pupils are Being Wrongly Excluded Over their Hair. I'm Trying to End This Discrimination." *Guardian*, 25 February, 2020.

Dabiri, Emma. *Don't Touch My Hair*. London: Penguin, 2019.

Dabiri, Emma, interview by Matt Elton. "Why Black Hair Matters." BBC History Extra Podcast. 05 08, 2019.

Darwin, Charles. *The Descent of Man*. London: John Murray, 1871.

Darwin, Charles. *The Origins of the Species*. London: John Murray, 1859.

Fanon, Franz. *Black Skin, White Masks*. New York: Grove Press, 1967.

Turner, John G. "The Great White God." In The Mormon Jesus: A biography, 249, 35. Harvard University Press, 2016.

"Genesis 4." In *The Bible*: Authorized King James Version with Apocrypha, edited by Robert Carroll and Stephen Prickett, 4–5. Oxford: Oxford World Classics, n.d.

Ikard, David H. "Rejecting Goldilocks: The Crisis of Normative White Beauty for Black Girls." In *Blinded by the Whites: Why Race Still Matters in 21st-Century America*. Indiana University Press, 2013.

Kendall, Mikki. *Hood Feminism*. London: Bloomsbury, 2020.

Levy, Andrea. *Small Island*. London: Headline, 2004.

Mayes, Ernest M. "As Soft as Straight Gets: African American Women and Mainstream Beauty." Counterpoints, 1997: 85–108.

Black and British: A Forgotten History. BBC. Performed by David Olusoga, 2016.

Fighting for King and Empire: Britain's Caribbean Heroes. Produced by BBC. Performed by David Olusoga, 2015.

Patton, Tracey Owens. "Hey Girl, Am I More than My Hair?: African American Women and Their Struggles with Beauty, Body Image, and Hair." NWSA Journal (The Johns Hopkins University Press) 18, no. 2 (2006): 24–51.

Prentiss, Craig R. "Coloring Jesus: Racial Calculus and the Search for Identity in Twentieth-century America." Nova Religio: The Journal of Alternative and Emergent Religions 11, no. 3 (2008): 64–82.

Self-Made. Produced by Netflix, 2020.

Snook, Edit. "Beautiful Hair, Health, and Privilege in Early Modern England." Journal for Early Modern Cultural Studies (University of Pennsylvania Press) 15, no. 4 (2015): 22–51.

Stuart Hall, Bill Schwarz. *Familiar Stranger: A Life Between Two Islands*. London: Penguin, 2018.

Tulloch, Carol. "Moving Here: Migration Histories: Good Grooming and Reconstruction." Web Archive, 2013.

White, Nadine. "More Than a Haircut: Why Black Salons Are Needed More Than Ever After Lockdown." Huffington Post, 19 July 2020.

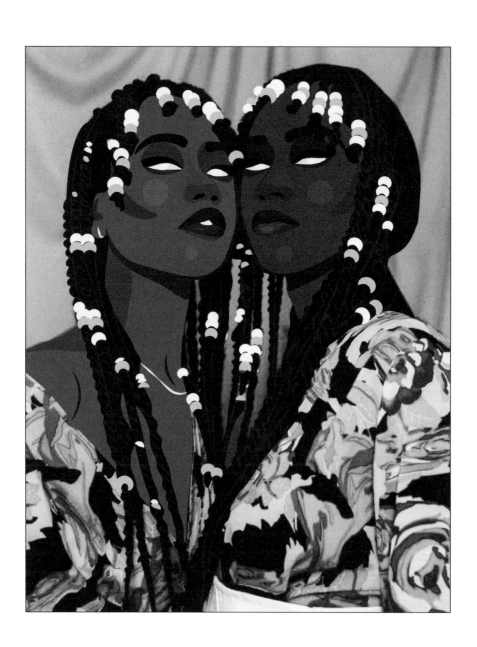

AUTHORS' NOTE

Saskia Calliste & Zainab Raghdo

The Black Lives Matter movement, particularly the 2020 protests and social media discourse that took place in the wake of the tragic murder of George Floyd, were the main impetus for this book. The discussions about racial justice were spurred by the video of the infamous killing, captured by a Black teenage girl, Darnella Frazier, on her mobile phone camera, as she was passing by with her cousin on a street in Minneapolis in May 2020. Later given a special Pulitzer award for her courage in recording the event, Darnella's video, which was shared on social media, led to international outrage, as well as mass protests in many countries for social justice. There followed a reexamination of the systemic racism at the heart of governments which place little value on Black lives. It also highlighted the negative perceptions and representations that many Western societies force on the Black body and hair, which are an integral part of that discussion.

Whilst skin colour is central to racial discrimination, it is not the only factor involved. Dark skin is not specific to African and Afro-Caribbean peoples, but Black hair is. It is this aspect of us that white society has used to label us as inhuman and unworthy for centuries. This discrimination continues to this day largely unchecked, because of the way that our kinky hair sets us apart.

Where reactions to our skin may differ, ridding ourselves of the kinks in our hair is an idea many of us seemed to agree on. We have all had negative experiences regarding our hair. If not, we have had a feeling for our hair, good or bad, that stemmed from the same prevailing narrative – that society does not represent Afro-textured hair as beautiful, proper, feminine or human.

We need to learn to give our hair the respect it deserves. That is what this book aims to do – to represent us in all our multifaceted, kinky-haired glory and create a space to discuss our experiences and say: "This is me!"

This book is also for anyone who has ever felt less worthy, undesirable or unloved because of the natural hair that grows out of their head. It aims to give a voice to those who have already experienced hair hate and remind us that we are never alone. It reminds us that we are a part of a beautiful, resilient, blooming global community of Black women, who embrace one another.

Despite the harsh truth it carries, this book is a celebration of Black women, their struggle, and how it has not stopped them from achieving greatness in their lives. We, as Black women, are usually left out of our own narrative, and when it comes to our hair, it's no different.

It seems to be acceptable for other cultures to wear dreadlocks, install a weave or get cornrows in their hair. While they are celebrated for being diverse or on-trend, these same culturally Black hairstyles often invoke criticism for the Black women who wear them, as being inappropriate in the workplace. No other race of women's hair carries the political weight that a Black woman's hair does, and we are tired of dealing with this burden. It is time to let it go.

From the diverse range of inspiring women we have had the absolute pleasure of interviewing, together, we are unapologetically reclaiming our narrative so that Black women and girls will no longer feel they are alone with the challenges of having Black hair.

Read these first-hand experiences, learn from the wisdom they reveal and, most importantly, love who you are.

NAMED FOR HER

Sheer.
Black.
Laddered.
Woven tight.
Into cornrows.
Ear to ear.
Forehead to nape.
Sectioned like a hot-cross bun.
Parted to show a caramelled brown surface
where the sun works with hair grease to
moisten the curly edges that shape her forehead,
brightening her face from matt to slightly shiny.

"That's my mum's face you have there."
I grinned and silently thanked Granny for being beautiful.

— Kadija Sesay

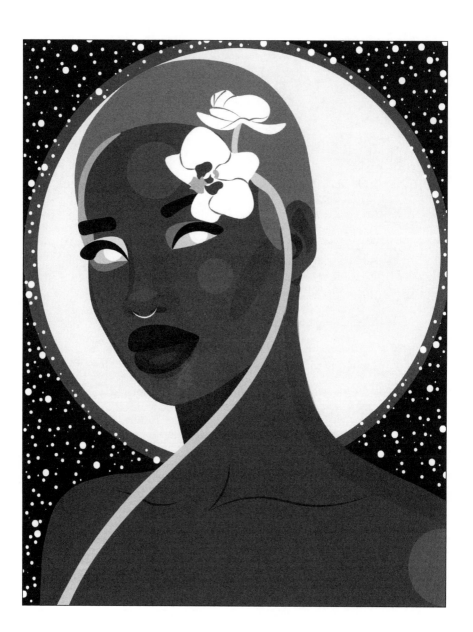

HER HAIR STORIES

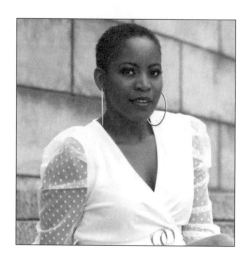

ANNIKA ALLEN

Annika Allen is the co-owner of entertainment platform The Black Magic Network and co-founder of the Black Magic Awards – a show created to honour and celebrate "extraordinary and inspirational" women of colour who have paved the way in various fields. She also works in Diversity & Inclusion for Barclays.

Annika has over 15 years of experience in the communications and marketing industry, leading on projects for brands such as Google UK, Universal and Skype that have delivered solid results and innovative experiences strategically devised to grow, inspire and entertain. Listed as one of the most inspirational Black British females in an article in *The Metro*, she is a sought-after speaker on business, diversity, social media and popular culture. Her entrepreneurial spirit, creative flair and go-getting attitude have enabled her to build businesses and brands and empower the next generation of creative talent through digital communications and entertaining and educational experiential events.

What was your go-to hairstyle as a child, and who used to do your hair?

I'm a twin – so my mum would end up doing our hair in two plaits. Mum would only do it if it were something basic, so little doobie plaits or up in a bun, nothing creative. Then a lady called Shirley, who lived on our local estate, used to braid it when we needed our hair in cornrows. And these were the times when people were burning the ends off cornrows. Having our hair braided in cornrows was probably our go-to hairstyle.

Who was your hair inspiration growing up? Did you struggle to find Black hair inspiration?

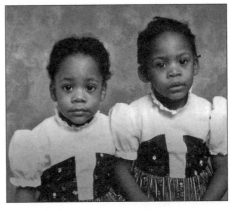

Luckily, I wasn't one of those people who was bothered that my hair had to look a certain way – it came as I got older. So, when I was a child – say, under 10 – I didn't think that much about my hair. It was just, "OK, I need to get it braided", and I'd be off out to play. Because I'm a twin, my sister and I loved *Tia & Tamera* and *Sister, Sister*, and we thought, "We'd love to look like them!" It was always [Black] American people because, aside from immediate family, you never really saw British Black people in the limelight. You'd think their hair looks amazing because a lot of people were wearing weaves on TV or in the spotlight. Most of my family have really lovely hair. Some of my family are Jamaican-Chinese, and some of them have got great, healthy, long natural hair, so I was always quite envious of their hair – growing down to their bottom and all flowing, and my hair was never going to grow like that.

Who are the Black female role models in society, and how do they differ from the role models you had growing up?

The beauty of today is that we can see the diversity of Black beauty and Black hair. Whether it's looking at Instagram or TV, movies and magazine stars and thinking, I like what they're doing. I think that's what's changed – we actually have the capacity to see the depth and breadth of Black hair, which we didn't when I was a kid and a teenager. When I was a teen, you had to have your hair in a weave, or you'd have your hair permed, whereas today, it's a lot more acceptable to have your natural hair. So, when I look at people like Lupita Nyong'o and her low hair and striking beauty and see stars now with bald heads, low hair, Afro hair, it's unapologetic.

At what age were you made to feel that your hair was different? Tell us about that experience, what it felt like and how you navigated that?

My school was predominantly white in the West Midlands, so I always knew that my hair and features weren't like everyone else around me. But lucky for me, I come from a Jamaican family that is very loud, very confident in who they are. If something looks good, they're telling you; if something doesn't look good, they're telling you. So being confident in who I am in general helped me not think about the difference between my hair and European

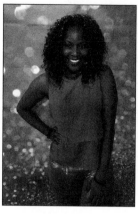

hair. And at school, my friends thought we were the "cool" friends. After PE in the changing rooms, I always knew I couldn't quickly wash my hair like the other girls, but it didn't make me feel any different.

What age were you when you started to make your own hair decisions? What were those decisions, and why did you choose the style you did?

When we were 12 or 13, my sister and I went to America to visit an aunt. In America, everybody had their hair permed – that was the style. I remember us getting our hair permed and my mum being upset when she saw us. As a teen, we started making our own decisions about what we would and wouldn't do with our hair. I probably wouldn't have done it in hindsight because my hair is quite fine in texture – when it was permed, it was quite thin and lifeless. Obviously, you do things to make it look cute, but it wasn't the best thing for my natural hair. I've been a bit of a chameleon with my hair. I've had a short weave, I've had a long weave, I've had burgundy, blonde – I'll just do anything. I think that's the confidence I have in Afro hair and beauty now, to do whatever, whenever I want. I work at Barclays bank – my day job at the moment – and I remember when I was going to start, I had my hair in four locs in crochet braids. I debated whether I should change my hair before starting work, as it might not be an appropriate hairstyle for a corporate company. And I then thought, nah, this is me; they're going to see a bunch of different hairstyles while I'm there because I never keep my hair the same style, so I want them to see me and be myself. I think probably a few years back, that wouldn't have been a choice because before you even started in the workplace, they probably would have told you to change your hairstyle before the interview.

Do you have any experiences where your hair had a major effect on something in your life?

My hair now – I cut it short in the first lockdown – I noticed there was a bald patch in the middle of my head. I don't know if it's a combination of being hormonal after having a baby or possibly stress with going back to work after maternity leave and being in lockdown, but there was a big hand-sized bald patch, and I didn't like it. So, I was wearing wigs and stuff to cover it. I was like, I don't want to continue wearing wigs and never wear my natural hair, so the doctor suggested iron tablets to help, and my partner was like, "Why not just cut it off?"

I called up a hairdresser I trusted and told her to come round my house and cut my hair, and she cut it really low. I was scared to take a pic and show people at first, but I just had to bite the bullet and do it, and I think it's definitely been the best thing. This is all me. I'd say that was probably the most eye-opening thing for me. And a lot of people have said this is the best style you've ever had.

I think I'm still learning about how to look after my hair. I'll talk to friends who have been on a natural hair journey, and they'll be like: use liquids, use oils, use creams. I've made my own cream out of shea butter and other oils to get into natural products rather than shop-bought products. I'm just being more mindful of the kinds of things I put in my hair and on my body and also being mindful of these things for my daughter. I do a lot more stuff at home now, trying to be a lot more conscious about my hair and having my natural hair allows me to do that. It's a journey that I'm slowly enjoying being on.

What do you think about how brands situate themselves in the narrative of Black hair? What more do you think could be done?

One of the things we've been deceived about all these years regarding hair products is that we have to use a specific product. However, white people could use certain products for Black hair if their hair's really coarse. Black women can use certain products marketed at Caucasians because maybe their hair is finer. So, I'm trying to learn more about what's good and what's bad to use on our hair.

I think it's good that we're seeing Afro hair products in some mainstream shops now, but they don't market that these products are available there, so sometimes these products can end up getting pulled from the shelves because maybe customers aren't buying those products. How can you buy something that you don't know is there? It's a shame that so many of the companies that used to be Black-owned initially have been bought by some of the bigger companies that don't necessarily care about us as consumers – they're not good at marketing the product or really engaging the Black community when it comes to their product.

In terms of haircare, I think Luster's the only one that's Black-owned now, that sits alongside L'Oréal and African Pride, which is a shame. But what's good now is that more and more beauty brands are coming up and making products and marketing them towards us because of the internet and access to some of the ingredients. I think that's beautiful to see because I'd definitely prefer to buy from an indie supplier, someone I know has made it from love and knows all of the ingredients in there, rather than one of the big players. They probably have ingredients in there that aren't good for hair in the first place.

But I don't think there are many companies that do enough to engage with us as consumers and engage with us as a community. I remember a few years ago when Shea Moisture had Black women build the brand and put money into it and then did an advert that either didn't have any Black women in it at all or didn't have any brown or dark-skinned women in the advert and there was an uproar about it. I remember thinking, well, actually, you are what you are today because of the money from the Black community, and this is what you do. What happened with George Floyd put the lens on the global Black diaspora community, so more brands are getting behind it, and some are just jumping on the bandwagon; time will tell if their efforts are authentic or not. When I hear people say today that they were excluded from school because they couldn't have dreads or a particular style or that their natural hair is too big, those things make my blood boil. How can you tell somebody, particularly when it comes to their natural hair, that their hair is too big or to get it under control? Now there's the Halo Code, the UK's first Black hair code for schools and workplaces that champions the rights of staff and students to embrace all Afro-hairstyles. There's also been the celebration of World Afro Day, so that's been amazing, with people pioneering Afro hair and championing it.

What do you think of the differences between the way Black men and Black women are treated in society when it comes to standards of beauty?

I don't think Black men are judged as much for their hairstyles as women are. And I think Black men judge a lot of women when it comes to their hair. This baffles me because I think many of them grew up with sisters and mums and saw what they were doing with their hair. So, I don't know why they're so judgemental, particularly if a woman's wearing a weave or a wig, even women wearing the Ghanaian things. Patterns and

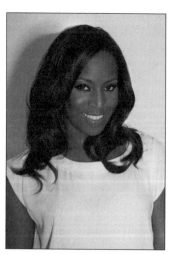

styles are a lot sexier these days than they were a few years ago, but ultimately our hair isn't the same as white people's hair, so we have to wear these things to help keep in the moisture and help it stay nice when we're sleeping. These are all things they saw growing up, but they don't want their partner or wife wearing that as they get older. I think that's probably the most hurtful thing when it comes to Black men and the difference between Black men and women and hair. For men, it's less maintenance – we're the ones who have to spend a lot of time in the hairdressers, probably more than they would in the barbershop. My partner takes his hair very seriously – he has to go to the barbers, so some men take their grooming very seriously. But one of the things I don't like is the comparison – like if Black men compare Black women to what white women do to their hair. It's comparing apples and pears: they're not the same, so don't compare the two; just appreciate your woman's beauty in whatever form that comes in.

What more do you think needs to be done to empower Black women, particularly regarding hair and beauty?

Even though there are platforms now for us to see Black hair and beauty, I still think the mainstream media doesn't highlight Black beauty enough. As Black women we have to battle mentally with the images that we see in the media. When we're presented with what beauty looks like, it's never us a lot of the time, so we have to be strong in mind and spirit to combat that. I know that my sisters and the Black women that I see are beautiful and diverse, and there's not one standard of beauty for us, even if that's what the media are showing us. I think it's about instilling that in ourselves and the next generation and particularly little children – especially now because the next generation will only know being on social media. The selfies and the posing provide more pressure to be constantly looking good, and observing other people and what they look like and comparing each other.

I think the next generation will have a harder time with that, so I think it's definitely just instilling in ourselves and each other that we are beautiful, just championing Black beauty in all its forms. So, if you're an editor of a magazine, it's making sure there's diversity in the publication. If you're in advertising, it's giving opportunities to Black voices to be seen and heard in these spaces. It's about people paving the way and sending the elevator down to bring Black people into these spaces, but also making everything normal. So it's normal to have Afro hair and be like that in the workplace. With what's happened in the last year in the pandemic, we'll never go back to working with everyone in the office, so people will be more comfortable with the skin they're in. I think working from home has allowed businesses to see people in their home environments; if you wanted to throw on a head wrap or haven't had a chance to do your hair because there are no hairdressers open, it's like, well, this is me, why would you go back to having to hide yourself? Be bold, be you, be authentic and don't be boxed in. The veil's been lifted, and that has been one of the beauties of being in these difficult times. For most of us, it's allowed us to be ourselves. That's one of the reasons that I started the Black Magic Awards, which is where we celebrate phenomenal Black British talent, because there are so many people who say that we don't see any role models, or if they do, it's still people in the US. But there are so many amazing Black British men and women in the UK doing so many amazing things.

When you're in that room and feel the sisterhood, the brotherhood, and hear those inspiring stories, it's such a motivating and uplifting experience. This year has allowed more of us to see each other, be kind to each other and be happy within ourselves.

What advice would you give to your younger self today? Or what do you wish your younger self had known, that you know today?

I would say anything in life is possible. When it comes to hair and beauty, I remember when I was 20 or 21, and I entered Miss Jamaica UK. When I was going to the training to meet other contestants, I'd often wear a hat on my head, or my hair was in braids. None of the other contestants thought that I would be winning. Because I was very relaxed when it came to my looks and a bit tomboyish, and I was rubbish with my hair. Luckily, a friend of mine who was good with hair came to me before the contest and said, "What do you want to do with your hair?" I knew the beauty standard was straight hair, so I thought, let me play the game, I need to have straight hair. So she pressed it straight, and she put in bonding extensions and straightened it. And I always remember walking into the venue and everyone looking at me, thinking, you look really different. On that day, I ended getting a prize for best smile, most aware of Jamaican knowledge, history and culture. I ended up winning, being crowned Miss Jamaica UK. So, it just reminded me of the power of hair and beauty and of not being afraid to change things up as long as you're comfortable. Because there is power in hair and beauty, the way we look and being confident in that power. I would say to my younger self: continue to be confident in the power of your melanin and Black beauty, and find strength in that.

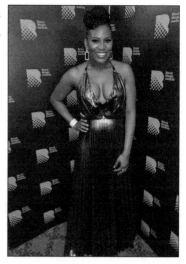

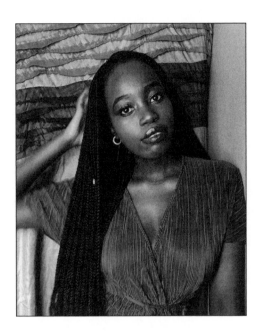

EVA ANEK

Eva Anek is an East Londoner born to Ugandan immigrant parents. She graduated with a BA Degree in Economics and Management from the University of Portsmouth. She currently works in financial services, and is an experienced business analyst with a demonstrated history of working in Information Technology and services. She is now working in her desired industry of luxury fashion, as she is an accountant for Prada. Alongside working for the fashion brand, she is studying towards her accounting qualifications, and hopes to be a fully qualified Chartered Accountant within the next three years.

What was your go-to hair style as a child, and who used to do your hair?

I've always had thick, natural hair and my lovely mum was my hairdresser. She used to tie it up in two cute little bunches, and when I got a little bit older, she used to cornrow it and then she started braiding my hair with expressions and I used to hate it because of the pain. When you're sitting in between her legs and she's braiding your hair, you don't want to say it's too tight, but it was too tight. My mum used to relax my hair too, can't forget about that, so

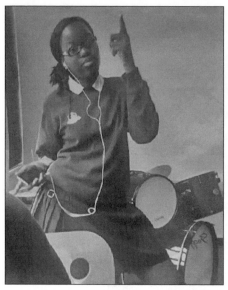

when I got to about 15, I decided to start wearing weave. A middle part of my leave out was really short because all of my relaxed hair broke off, but I still wanted to straighten it a little bit to make sure it blended in. Then I started wearing the half-wigs because I wanted to try that, so this was when I had the front of my hair out and I straightened it every single day to blend it in, breaking it off as well because I wasn't using any heat protection. I didn't care, I just wanted to make sure that the wig looked good. Then when I got to college, I had to cut all my hair off, and that's when I started wearing wigs full time, because I don't have the head shape for short hair. I was wearing wigs up until my second year of university then I was like, "OK, let's try braids again." I didn't like it, so I went back to wigs. If I didn't have a wig, I didn't feel good. In 2020, I decided to start embracing more natural hairstyles, so braids, twists and my natural hair.

Who was your hair inspiration growing up? Did you struggle to find Black hair inspiration?

I didn't have hair inspiration when I was young. Obviously, you look at your mum as the first beautiful woman in your life. My mum can rock short hair, so she always had short hair, but short hair wasn't for me. I always wondered when I was younger, "Why don't I see people with natural hair?" I just didn't see it, and this was the early 2000s when I really started noticing that I don't see natural hair ever. My eldest sister, about 10 years older than me, she always had relaxed hair so maybe that kind of inspired me to force my mum to relax my hair too, because I saw it on her.

I never had a person that I wanted my hair to look like until I got to my teen years and that's when I fell in love with Naomi Campbell and I was like, "Yep – that hair right there – that straight middle parting, long luscious hair." I came to that realisation when I was seventeen and that's when I started with straight, long middle parting wigs for six years straight. I thought her look was the epitome of beauty because I always saw her look celebrated. And I didn't see any Black models on the cover of magazines when I was younger. I don't know if this was ignorance but I feel like this celebration of Black beauty is very recent. When I was young, I couldn't go on the internet and see a dark skin girl getting all the love. People used to say horrible things to me when I was in school.

Who are the Black female role models in society, and how do they differ from the role models you had growing up?

In society now, my role models are Issa Rae, TV producer, actress, goddess everything. I really look up to her because, first of all, I don't see people that look like her in Hollywood and I think she has everyday beauty that me and you can recognize and see ourselves in her. I can't necessarily see myself in someone that looks like Jorja Smith, or Maya Jama. Issa is awkward, she's quirky, and the fact that she has made it to that level gives me hope, even though I have no desire to produce my own TV show. She is setting the precedent and breaking down barriers to make me feel like anyone can do it and she shows that the way she looks doesn't hold her back. Because, I'm pretty sure in the past, the way Black women have looked has held them back in their careers in many industries.

Michelle Obama – read her book and fell in love with her – I love intelligent women. I think she's extremely inspirational, and extremely smart, and it shows that women can do it. People, to this day, call her all types of names and she doesn't let that faze her because she's going to be who she's going to be, and she is a powerhouse to me. I'm mainly pointing out American women. Yes, America has a lot of problems, but America is way more diverse than the UK. That's why I'm inspired by more American women than British women. Serena Williams is the third most inspirational one to me. I'm not a sports person, but because my parents are really into tennis, we were watching Serena and Venus when we were small. To see where she's come from and how she is today – everything that she's had to deal with – and how that did not stop her. How can you *not* find that inspirational? She's an icon.

When you were younger who did you used to look up to?

When I was younger it was mostly pop stars, which is weird because I don't really care what these people are doing now. I used to look up to Rihanna and Beyoncé because I thought they were really beautiful women who could sing, and I wanted to be in the music videos with them. I don't know why I identified with them, I just wanted to be *that* girl, but I was never *that* girl. When you're eight years old you're not thinking about colourism or features, you're just identifying with any Black girl in any group.

When you were young, what beauty standards did you associate with being beautiful and how do they differ from today?

Beauty to me today? I feel like there's no definition, personally. I feel like confidence is beauty to me. When I see a confident woman walking down the street, I don't care what she's wearing, I don't care what she looks like. That was not the story when I was younger. I used to think having lighter skin was beautiful. I used to think that having luscious long hair was beautiful. Funnily enough, I didn't think being skinny was beautiful because I was quite skinny when I was younger, and people used to tell me to eat. But definitely the long hair, the light skin, that was gold in my eyes, but I didn't take it as far as wanting to bleach or do any of that, but I would say that I did really take it into consideration when I started to wear weaves or wigs.

Today I just love confidence. I love seeing Black women confident within their skin, I love seeing Black women confident in their features, I love seeing Black women confident in their hair, however they decide to style their hair.

What's your experience with featurism? It's not spoken about the way colourism is, but it is something that has always been there in the background.

I'll speak for fashion in particular. I feel like the Black models that they do choose have features that are not considered typical African features, such as a wider nose. Their features are more Eurocentric and that's why I always see the same kind of women. They tend to be from East Africa, like Sudan. That image will be used in high fashion even though their skin may be dark but their features will still be Eurocentric. I don't know if we're moving forward or not. Don't get me wrong, I love to see dark skin women on these covers, but am I seeing someone like Michaela Coel on these covers? No.

At what age were you made to feel like your hair was different? Tell us about that experience, what it felt like and how you navigated that?

Oh, I realized when I was young, at primary school. Six or seven years old. Because I was thinking to myself, "Why can't I just go to school with my hair out?" It was always at the back of my mind: "Why does it need to be in braids?" In primary school, the boys would ask: "Why don't you ever show your real hair?" They would say other mean things as well but I never had an answer to that question because I didn't know. I just had to deal with it, because I wasn't going to ask my mum to take my hair out of the braids. People used to try to pull the little ribbons out to see if my hair would fall downward like theirs, but they were actually pulling my hair. So I just internalized it and I continued like that throughout secondary school. I never showed my real hair in secondary school, or in college. When I was at uni, that's when I started embracing my natural hair. People would be like, "Oh you have such long hair," and I would just tell them, that it doesn't matter. I've always been taught by society that my hair had to be covered in some way.

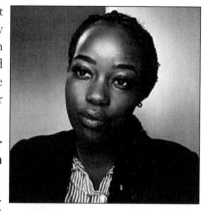

Have there been any times when your experiences with your hair have had a major effect on your life?

Yes. My hair falls out when I'm stressed. There was a point at uni during my final year, when I was doing things last minute and working under pressure, and my hair was in a bun. I went to check the back and I didn't feel much hair there and I realized I had a bald spot. That is when I started to take my health more seriously because I didn't want to be walking around with bald spots or having to wear a wig to cover it. That's when I started to love my hair as well.

At secondary school if a girl relaxed her hair and it was short, the girls would say to her, "What happened to your hair? It just broke off. Your hair's disgusting." I didn't want to be dealing with that, so that's why I made sure no one saw my natural hair in school. That's when I was most ashamed of my hair. I didn't want anyone to make fun of it. What I did have though, was other Black girls making fun of my skin tone.

What do you think about the division between Black girls based on how they wear their hair? Do you think it's still going on?

Back in the day, it was war. Things have gotten better but I think that it's still relevant. Maybe because I'm not in school I don't see it so much because the real world isn't as cliquey, but on social media there's a clique of the girls with the weave or the lace fronts who section themselves off, then those with the natural hair are off somewhere else. It's still there today. Is it conscious? I don't know, but it's something I would want to see broken down, because hair shouldn't be that serious. Hair shouldn't divide us. Hair should be fun.

When it comes to our hair, we Black women can sometimes tear each other down. It's like those who wear weaves are trying to be something that they're not. As if they're trying to dilute their Blackness or hide it. I think Black girls are told that they have to be authentically Black otherwise they get judged.

When you are at work, how do you wear your hair?

When I'm at work my hair is mainly in braids – it's convenient. I don't need to think about it. I get the most compliments when my hair is in braids. I've never had a negative experience with my hair in the workplace, not even when I wear a wig. Nor with my natural hair either. I'm quite surprised because my industry is fashion. It's all about looks. I'm thankful that I haven't experienced that because I wouldn't know how to react.

What do you think about how brands situate themselves in the narrative of Black hair? What more do you think could be done?

Brands need to recognize that Black beauty comes in all different shades, shapes and sizes, so can we please not have the same look over and again? I'm 25 years old and the images of Black women given to us are the same as when I was young. I think that's ridiculous. That's why I'm thankful for platforms like Instagram because on there I can see the Black girl that's more punk rock being celebrated, because people need to understand there isn't only one skin tone, or one hairstyle when it comes to Black. There isn't a mould of a specific Black girl that every Black girl needs to fit into. Just let us live.

What advice would you give to your younger self today? Or what do you wish your younger self had known, that you know today?

Don't feel so ashamed because you have nothing to feel ashamed about when it comes to your looks. Stop worrying because life is life. It will take you wherever it will take you. I used to be so fixated on the future, thinking I would have my life sorted by a certain age. Just be more confident and embrace the

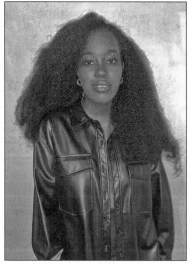 person that you are. Just be at peace with yourself.

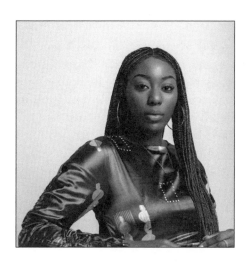

ANITA ASANTE

Anita is the founder of BLANC. NOIR, an independent strategic global brand relationship building consultancy specialising in beauty, fashion, lifestyle and music. She loves people and her purpose in life is to uplift ethnic minorities and push them to the forefront of everything she does. "I'm all about pushing forward Black voices and inspiring highly successful brand partnerships specifically for the BIPOC community that makes a positive difference".

Anita has worked with clients such as Adidas, Target, Ben & Jerry's, YouTube, *Nataal Magazine* (an African global media brand) and the world renowned music festival AfroPUNK (which attracts 130,000+ creators annually who express their alternative narratives on identity through music, style, arts and culture) for years now with the main goal to push the culture forwards in all ways, always. Anita is also a natural hair enthusiast and born out of her personal journey is currently using her knowledge of her own hair needs to fill in the gap of the UK hair industry market with a scalp and hair care essentials product brand set to launch in Q4, 2021.

What was your go-to hairstyle as a child, and who used to do your hair?

When I first read this question, I let out a little chuckle because boy oh boy, the hairstyles I used to rock as a child... well let's just put it this way, I was no wallflower that's for sure. I'm of Ghanaian heritage and my mum used to be a hairdresser – had a lovely little salon in Tottenham – and so when I think back on it, she definitely unleashed her creativity on my older sister and I when it came to our hair. Her go-to style for me though was African threading.

I remember vividly going to primary school with my hair neatly threaded up and actually funnily enough being told I had "worms" growing out of my head by some of the kids at school – charming! But it didn't bother me so much to be honest as when my hair was in this style, I was able to wear my favourite white ribbon tied into a bow and that's all that mattered because with that bow, I felt like I was the bee's knees.

When my hair wasn't threaded, it was either in big chunky doo doo plaits accompanied by all kinds of colourful hair baubles or colourful 1B mid-length braids. I don't remember ever having my hair just out as a child, it was always in some sort of protective style.

Who was your hair inspiration growing up? Did you struggle to find Black hair inspiration?

Truthfully, I didn't have any. Growing up, I can't remember thinking that anyone who was Black and famous at the time had hair that I could relate to. It was always either super long and straight (think Aaliyah), in a blonde-coloured Afro (think Scary Spice Mel B), in super long braids (think Moesha) or there were the girls with super sleek shiny hair on the Dark and Lovely perm kits you saw at the Black hair shop. I didn't really see natural hair 4A – 4C hair growing up aside from that of my cousins or friends and even they at times more often than not had succumbed to the creamy crack in order to get that look and be that girl. My mum never allowed me to perm my hair and during my teenage years (when I took over doing my own 4A hair) it was tough to be able to figure out how to style and take care of my hair.

Who are the Black female role models in society, and how do they differ from the role models you had growing up?

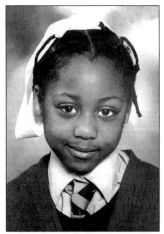

My peers. I just love the natural hair movement that has sprung up especially over the last few years. It truly warms my heart and as a naturalista, I get so much info from Instagram and discovering all of these ways to care for our hair. The difference from what it was like growing up, is that society is far more embracing of natural hair and all of our different types of curl patterns within that and provides the right information as to how best to care, treat and nourish our hair to essentially keep it flourishing.

When you were young, what beauty standards did you associate with being beautiful, and how do they differ today?

That creamy crack! It had to be relaxed hair most definitely. The images of the young girls on the Dark and Lovely perm kit boxes definitely had an impact on what I saw as beautiful. I equated the shiny sleek hair to beauty and if you had anything but that, then you weren't deemed as desirable. Thankfully, I soon grew out of that and today, it's a complete 360° turnaround. I'm super grateful that I was never allowed to perm my hair and was able to see and be able to manipulate my hair in its natural state.

At what age were you made to feel like your hair was different? Tell us about that experience, what it felt like and how you navigated that?

When I started to straighten my hair to achieve that sleek look and it all broke and became heat damaged. I think I was around the age of 14 and I continued to straighten it until the damage breakage became really bad so then I moved to braids.

What age were you when you started to make your own hair decisions, what were those decisions, and why did you choose the style you did?

I was 14, I believe in Year 9 and one day I just woke up and decided right I want to start doing my own hair. My mum fought me on it but I was super persistent and after a while she relented and I was free. No more doo doo plaits etc., I literally for the first time in my life had control of my own hair and I was so excited. I bought a straightener (my parents would not buy me the GHD's so I had to settle for Remington's, go figure) and thus began the beginning of the end of my healthy head of hair. Ha! I straightened it to death, always scraped it up into a high pineapple with a side sweep, because that was the it-girl style at the time and pretty soon, unsurprisingly, my hair began to break but I kept on straightening it as I just loved that look and I didn't care what it cost to achieve it.

Do you have any experiences where your hair had a major effect on something in your life?

When I started wearing braids and discovered I suffered from a really irritated scalp and it would be dry, flaky and you could see the flakes through my braids. At one point I became really self-conscious about it, which in a way knocked my confidence a bit. I was able to treat it and is really what set me on my own journey to create my own scalp and hair care essentials line where my true discovery lay in the fact that the scalp is the extension of the skin in need of tender loving care, and ultimately the root to healthy hair. It's been quite a cathartic relief in knowing that what used to cause me so much angst has now proven to be a bigger blessing and I'm super excited to release these products into the world.

How do you wear your hair at work? Or for interviews? Has this changed over time?

I change my hair all the time! From wigs, jumbo braids, Senegalese twists, cornrows, locs, micro braids, ponies, beaded styles to my go-to natural slick back look, I've always kept it moving with the latest styles. I've also been pretty fortunate that for the most part, my career has been in the creative industry: fashion and beauty and then today it's expanded into the music and live experience space which has allowed me to be quite expressive with my hair and so I never really felt pressured to have my hair in a certain way.

I also run my own consultancy business now so it makes it easier to set the hair agenda from the offset. Although in saying that, and quite a funny story, a couple of years ago I was in Paris for a festival, AfroPUNK, and I obviously had my hair made up for the occasion – think beads, gold wires, everything. I was also interviewing at the time (long story short, I had lived in New York for five years and was making the move back to London so had been applying for roles around that time) and right before heading to the airport, I received an email from my potential prospective employer (which thinking back to it oddly was in the tech space – I wanted to try something new I guess) that I had a second round interview which would take place whilst I was in Paris and I remember acutely thinking, "Oh shoot, what am I going to do about my hair?" I literally grabbed a wig from the side table and stuffed it into my suitcase thinking I'll deal with that later. Fast forward a couple of days, I'm desperately trying to fit a wig over my beaded braided head and my boyfriend is looking at me like what on earth are you doing and I distinctly remember saying, "I have to look professional so help me get this wig on". I have the interview and it goes well (didn't get the job in the end but hey ho, it certainly wasn't meant to be) and once all is said and done I get up, catch a glimpse of myself in the mirror and all the while I've been sitting there over zoom with my wig on and my braided beads coming out underneath my wig – it was a mess. I was so annoyed and more so at myself and literally vowed from that day forward, that I would never ever do that to myself again – try and dim who I really am to fit in and fortunately from then, I haven't had to. I turn up to meetings authentically, more often than not with my natural slicked back style which I love and has been my go-to over the last couple of years – I love braids too

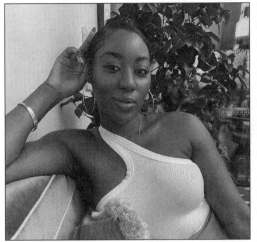

but historically, I haven't been able to wear them as often as I like due to scalp issues but I'm tackling that day by day with my brand. Stay tuned!

What part does your hair play in your life today? What in your "hair story" helped shape that?

A huge role in my life. My hair is truly a big part of my identity and it makes up a huge part of who I am. In the same way I approach fashion and my "lewks", I look at hair as the ability to change your mood, your vibe, your entire being. When I decided a couple of years ago to fully be a natural babe (spurred on by an irritated scalp) and by that I mean, not wearing wigs day to day and whilst I would rock braids on occasion, that could not become my go-to due to scalp irritation, it truly revolutionized my life. I became so acutely aware of the ingredients I was using in my shampoo/conditioners and general hair care regimen and I took a vested interest in how to properly care for my scalp and hair, staying away from the silicone laden products that did more harm than good to my scalp and hair despite their 'efficacy' claims. I studied up, increased my knowledge base around my hair and even embarked on some DIY home treatments to fill in the gaps of what I think is missing in the market. I take pride in the fact that I'm able to wear my hair in its natural state. It's made me so much more confident in just feeling beautiful in my own skin without the need for all of the added extras.

What do you think about how brands situate themselves in the narrative of Black hair? What more do you think could be done?

Erasure is such a key word for me in this conversation. Black women in particular spend almost six times more on hair products than white women do but are often overlooked and left out of the conversation. That's slowly beginning to change as the big-player brands are seeing how much money can be made by capturing the Black woman's attention and so we are starting to see an influx of marketing geared towards us as they realize the power of the Afro community. The problem is, they don't understand our needs and so inadvertently we continue to get overlooked and marginalized.

What do you think of beauty products such as skin-lightening creams?

Abhor them. To be honest it makes me really sad when I see people who feel the need to use skin-lightening creams. Our skin colour is so beautiful, so melanated and it should be celebrated. In the same way that we have regulations around certain medications, skin-lightening creams should be treated in the same way. They promote the notion that lighter skin is best which is incredibly damaging.

Can you easily find beauty products which suit your skin tone?

Fenty Beauty certainly made it easier.

What more do you think needs to be done to empower Black women, particularly regarding hair and beauty?

Listen to Black women. Don't ignore our needs or our wants and don't erase our identity by proliferating Eurocentric ideals of beauty as the ideal standard. Black women are beautiful, our hair is truly our crowning glory and similarly to the strands on our head, we are delicate so treat us with kindness and most importantly make a space that allows for our voice to be heard.

What advice would you give to your younger self today? Or, what do you wish your younger self had known, that you know today?

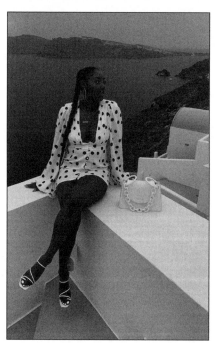

Trust your gut and just do it. Seriously! And if it scares you, then do it even more so.

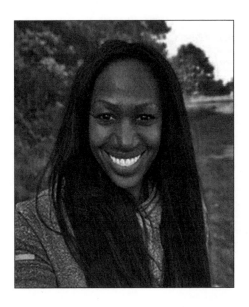

CAROLINE BLACKBURN

Caroline Blackburn is currently completing her Master's in Education, specialising in ages three to seven years. She is passionate about children's books and is focusing on encouraging diversity and inclusion in storybooks within this age range. At the age of one, Caroline was adopted by a white family, and as they travelled around the world, she was often the only Black child in her school. Although her family educated her, there was a lack of ethnic books available for her to read. Her mother finally found Caroline her first Black book at the age of nine.

Previously, Caroline was an International Bobsleigh athlete for Great Britain, selected for the Olympics in 2002. Like any top professional sportsperson, Caroline experienced her share of injuries, which prompted her to pursue her sports injury and rehabilitation qualifications and complete a Bachelor of Science with Honours Degree in Sports Studies.

With over 15 years of experience in Sports Therapy, Caroline has owned Sports and Injury Clinics in England and France, and gained a distinguished reputation working with international athletes, celebrities and the general public. She has travelled around the world working at major sporting competitions and with high profile clients. She has inspired many people to pursue their goals and in France was the voice of supporting local businesses. She was also recognized for encouraging children in sport through motivational speaking.

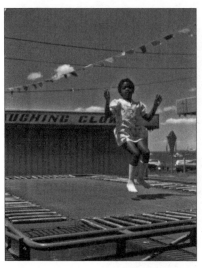

What was your go-to hairstyle as a child?

I had a short Afro, but always wanted it to be big. I was never completely happy with my hair. I felt that I looked like a boy, as my mum always kept it short for school, as it was easier to control. I remember my mum tugging at my hair with an Afro comb trying to control my hair. I was adopted by a white couple, and I remember they gave me a book when I was nine called *The Black Book of Beauty*. It was full of pictures of Black women with Afros, so that was the only style I knew.

Who was your hair inspiration growing up? Did you struggle to find Black hair inspiration?

When I was young, it was Diana Ross. I was so confused as to why my hair was growing up and out, and hers was long, thick and curly. When I was older, I admired Whitney Houston. I was inspired by both women because I always wanted thick, long, curly hair, that went down past my shoulders.

Who are the Black female role models in society, and how do they differ from the role models you had growing up?

Today, Michelle Obama is inspirational and approachable, and I admire Oprah Winfrey for what she has experienced and achieved. It was always models and singers as role models. We still have these like Beyoncé and Rihanna, who are very successful, but we now have Black women recognized in other industries: writers, designers, scientists.

When you were young, what beauty standards did you associate with being beautiful, and how do they differ today?

My mum did not encourage me to wear make-up, but I loved fashion. However, I lived in the countryside and was obsessed with sport, so I saw beauty in the athletes. I had posters on my wall of Olympians, Jackie Joyner-Kersee and Flo Jo (Florence Griffith Joyner) who used to wear very long nails and unique outfits on the track. To me, they were beautiful as they were glamorous and amazing athletes.

At what age were you made to feel like your hair was different? Tell us about that experience, what it felt like and how you navigated that?

I lived in Scotland in the countryside and was the only Black person within a large radius. So, I always knew my hair was different. Then when I moved down to Cheshire, again, I was the only Black person in my new school. It was when I was 16 years old, that I realized my hair could be different. I went to watch Wet, Wet, Wet, in Manchester with school friends, and when walking to the venue, I had never seen so many Black people in my life. I remember thinking, "How has she got straight hair, and I haven't?" On the way back from the concert, I asked my friends, "Could we stop off at a hairdresser?" My friends went in with me and I explained to the hairdresser that, "I wanted my hair to be 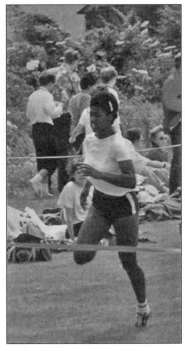 straight and could he style it?" The hairdresser said, "Yes, he could try." It is what you call relaxing." So, I went home, told my mum, and she said I would have to save up for it as it was expensive. I saved up the money, went back into Manchester, and they straightened my hair. I was happy with the style. However, I remember it being slightly painful, a burning feeling. I did not understand that it was a chemical treatment. My hair was not completely straight; it had a slight kink in it. Unfortunately, the relaxer only lasted roughly three weeks, and then it started to go very curly again, which really upset me. It was not until I moved to London, to go to university, that somebody introduced me to weaves. I was 21 by then, so it was a long time before I knew what a weave was.

What age were you were you when you started to make your own hair decisions?

I was 16. When shopping with my mum or friends, I would go into every hairdressers with a photo of a Black woman in the window, or if I saw a Black woman in the street, I would ask her, "Where did you get your hair styled?"

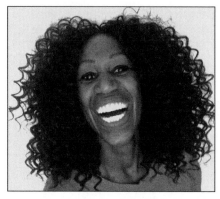

Did you have any experiences where your hair had a major effect on something in your life?

Yes, it was three years ago that I had my first encounter, when I went to work in recruitment. I had an interview, and my hair was Black, straight and long down my back. I got the job, so, I thought as I have a new job, I'd like a new hairstyle – something funky but still smart.

I drove all the way down to London to get my hair done by my old hairdresser and when I went into the office on the Monday, a few people in the office were complimentary, saying, "Oh, wow, that's amazing, it suits you." I sat amongst eight desks in a row. There were two managers, one was sitting beside me, and the Director, who was sitting nearby. He literally turned around to me and said, "Why have you got your hair like that? It looks ridiculous. You should have kept it straight." He said that in front of everybody. It was an open-plan office, with over fifty people in the room. I saw the people sitting behind and in front of me raise their eyes or snigger. It was a horrible experience, but I am quite stubborn and as I really liked this hairstyle, I was not going to change it. However, it did make me paranoid. I was constantly trying to calm it down when I was going to work by putting clips in it to pull it back off my face or putting a headband on, and then really fluffing it back up when I got home or got out the office door. That was the start of the snide comments; they thought that I was not looking professional enough. Now, I realize that I was being bullied and I feel it was discrimination.

Then more recently, I'd been attending a course at university, and when I went in with a much tighter curl style than before, I did notice a reaction from some of the teachers. I just ignored it at first, but I just did not have the confidence to keep it like that, so I decided to get it straightened again, ready for my school placement. I felt like I was going to get judged negatively again. I am still apprehensive about whether to go with curly hair or leave it straight in a school environment.

What do you think about how brands situate themselves in the narrative of Black hair? What more do you think could be done?

There are plenty of Black hair shops with a variety of products and styles at affordable prices. However, I feel overwhelmed, as I do not know which product is right for me, especially as I am sporty and spend a lot of time in the water. So, when I go into the shops, I really need somebody that I can trust to say, "OK, this is what you want."

What about the skin-lightening creams?

When I visit the hair shops, the skin creams are the first thing you see at the counter. I would never use the creams, as I am happy with my skin colour and I feel there is no reason why I should change. I find it quite concerning that people feel they need to change their skin colour and do not understand the damage they can do.

What advice would you give to your younger self today? Or, what do you wish your younger self had known, that you know today?

My mum and dad did their best to find me books and talk about the history of Black people, including slavery. They did not go into detail, as they could see I would get upset. I still get upset learning about this period of colonial history, but I need to understand what happened. It is part of our collective history. I think that there is a debate around what age children need to be before the subject of slavery is discussed, but the subject cannot be avoided.

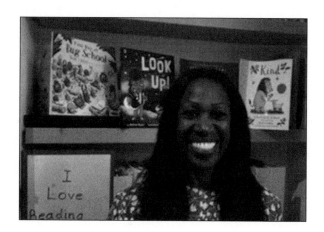

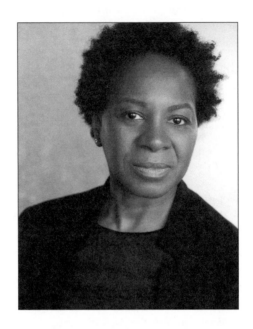

DOREENE BLACKSTOCK

Doreene Blackstock is a British actress, born and raised during the 60s, to Jamaican parents, in 2021's #CityOfCulture, Coventry. She describes herself as a #ModernDayGriot, who picked up her storytelling skills as a child while visiting relatives from Jamaica who brought stories of family back home, reggae music, Duppies and Anansi the spider Folklore, infused with rum, exotic fruits, sunshine and laughter.

Doreene is best known for her roles as Beatrice Effiong (Eric's Mum) in the Netflix hit TV Series, *Sex Education* and she's also known for her portrayal of DC Annie Reiss in *Wire in the Blood*. Her poem 'The Missing I in You' appears in the *Sista!* Anthology published by Team Angelica. She is currently writing her first full-length play, *Behind God's Back*.

What was your go-to hairstyle as a child, and who used to do your hair?

My mum always combed my hair. My dad attempted to do it once while mum was in the hospital giving birth to one of my siblings. It was an experience I'll never forget! I looked like Worzel Gummidge, the scarecrow, by the time he'd finished with it. My go-to hairstyles were two bunches or two plaits, with a parting straight down the middle.

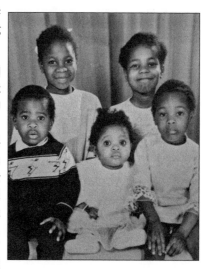

What age were you when you started to make your own hair decisions? What were those decisions, and why did you choose the style you did?

I was probably aged between 13 and 14 years old when I started to make decisions and choices about how I wanted my hair to look. I was influenced and inspired to try different styles by the other Black girls who attended my secondary school. There weren't many of us, but if one of us tried something new and it looked good, the others would follow.

Also, I was raised in the Pentecostal Christian faith. As a regular church attendee, I had plenty of opportunities to observe what other young Black women were doing with their natural hair, especially the women who visited from churches from cities like London, Birmingham, Nottingham and Leeds. My mum occasionally straightened my hair with a hot comb. That distinct smell of singed hair never leaves the memory. Chemically relaxing my hair was not an option for me. I was too young, and the church considered it sinful and vain, so I had to wait until I was 18 and at drama school. I relaxed my hair for years, a decision I would later regret, but at the time, I wanted to fit in. It was fashionable, it appeared to be so versatile, I wanted my Afro kinks to lay flat, it was manageable, or so it seemed until your relaxed hair got wet! To repair my hair, I went through a phase of plaiting it and adding beads, like Stevie Wonder on the cover album of *Hotter than July*. It looked great, my friends liked it, and my mum was very impressed because I did it all by myself. I'd go to school swishing my hair from side to side, and I thought it was fantastic.

Who was your hair inspiration growing up? Did you struggle to find Black hair inspiration?

My mum, aunts, cousins maybe? When I was growing up, there was very little or no inspiration for young Black women on how to wear their hair. You certainly didn't see any images in magazines or newspapers. Maybe on TV, Nina Baden-Semper (*Love Thy Neighbour*), Diahann Carroll (*Julia*). But these women wore wigs that represented the Caucasian aesthetic like most other actresses and Black celebrities at the time. Black music was inspirational, and high-profile artists such as Diana Ross, Aretha Franklin, Donna Summer and those big Afros were attractive and doable, but growing up in Coventry, inspiration for my hair was limited. There was a time (like most girls my age) when I was obsessed with Farrah Fawcett's hair! I have a horrendous photo of my hair curled like Farrah Fawcett's; I coaxed my Afro hair onto big curlers overnight, flicked it back and went out the next morning feeling good about my effort. My friends were very kind to me that day; even though it looked a mess and nothing at all like Farrah's hair, they said it looked nice.

Who are the Black female role models in society, and how do they differ from the role models you had growing up?

Michaela Coel is certainly a leading Black female role model, and then there is Cynthia Erivo, Noma Dumezweni, Marianne Jean-Baptiste – I could go on. Encouragingly, there is a long list of Black British female role models for today's Black women, young and old, and these women are not afraid to cut their hair and wear it short, natural and curly. These women represent strength and beauty. They bring the Black Afro aesthetic to life on and off-screen, and they are influential. Growing up in Coventry, I was related to most of the Black people I saw and knew. Our parents were the Windrush Generation. The only media references I had growing up were American. Even when Oprah first landed on the scene, her hair was straight.

Do you have any experiences where your hair had a major effect on something in your life?

Yes, the day I decided to cut my hair. When I entered the hairdressers salon, it

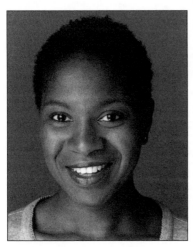

was relaxed, straight and long. I remember giving clear instructions to chop the lot! I'd had enough of subjecting my hair and scalp to caustic chemicals, and it was thinning. I had no idea the amount of damage that was being caused. Also, back in the day, maintaining and relaxing hair wasn't cheap. You couldn't buy the relaxer over the counter as you can now, and Black hairdressers were few and far between. You had to travel to get to a Black hair salon. As a struggling (freelance) Black actress, I had to prioritize other things. Straightening my hair was a luxury, so it had to go! I went back to Black, all-natural, all Afro and curly, and it paid off. It was a major game-changer for me. I even dyed it blonde, and the jobs came rolling in. My theatrical agents who represented me at the time loved it! I've never looked back.

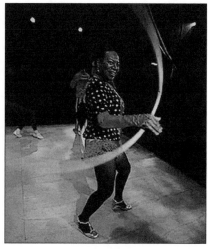

Netflix is fantastic, because they have all the top people there. And companies like The Royal Shakespeare Company – they are impeccable, because they make wigs all the time. There's no excuse now – if they want a Black woman to have straight hair and she's got natural hair, they can absolutely do it. More and more now they understand that. Because it's down to us at the end of the day, to – without apologies – just say, look, this is how I present. When I auditioned for the role, this is how I presented in the audition, and if you want me to do something else, let's all be creative. Because we're in the creative industries, let's all work together to get the image that we want. And I'm not afraid to walk away from something if they're insistent that my hair has to be straight. I can just say, "No, this job's not for me, it's for someone else."

There's this idea that if you don't comply, you won't get a job – that's a lie. I did what I wanted to do for me, because at the end of the day it's your talent. If you're the right person for the job, they're going to employ you regardless. So that was really empowering. And it was nice for me to be able to be a role model for other Black women. Especially younger Black women coming up in the industry. I was completely bald at one point. A bit like T'Nia Miller. It's very influential when you see other Black women doing it, you just go, "Yeah, I'm on the right path."

What part does your hair play in your life today?

Ultimately, I'm the only person responsible for my hair's health and maintenance. My Afro is versatile and easy to style. If I need to change it drastically for a character role or just for fun, I dye it or wear a wig. I'm proud of my Afro and what it represents: my African heritage/ancestry. My natural Afro hair tells the viewer what my idea of beauty is. When I was a young girl, that wasn't always the case. I choose how I wear my hair, and that's empowering.

What do you think about how brands situate themselves in the narrative of Black hair? What more do you think could be done?

Wow, when I was growing up, brands didn't cater to Black women for anything. Now brands have finally worked out that not only do we have money, but we also have lots of it, and we are hungry to spend it on any new product or thing that beautifies Black skin or manages our kinky hair. I think the more Black faces we see in advertising, the better. We need to see Black faces on product packaging, on the front cover of glossy magazines, featuring natural Afro hair in all its many forms, styles and beauty. Seeing influencers such as Michaela Coel, Letitia Wright, T'Nia Miller, wearing their natural hair, Chiney Bumps (Bantu knots), Afros, Box Braids etc.– this makes a difference. If I think a brand is for me and has been produced with me and my Black skin or hair in mind, I'll buy it, and I'm prepared to pay 'top dollar'. It's also important to support alternative, independent producers making healthy skin and hair products specifically for the Black market, like Big Hair + Beauty founder, Melissa Sinclair. We need to redirect wealth to brands made by Black owners who know the nature of our hair and how it behaves in all environments.

What do you think of the differences between the way Black men and Black women are treated in society when it comes to standards of beauty?

Multicultural, diverse Britain won't stand for it now, but Black beauty used to come down to shades of Blackness, and that's the ugly truth. When I left drama school and started auditioning for acting roles back in the 80s, #COLORISM was real. What gradient of Blackness determined what roles you were offered – complexion wars. Light skin acceptable; dark skin on our stages, TV screens and cinemas, not so much. It was evident that Black women

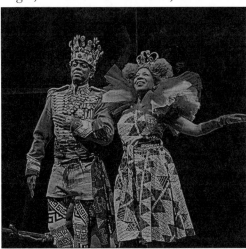

with lighter skin, acceptable (Caucasian) features and loose curly hair were considered more beautiful. They had more of a chance of being offered leading roles, especially in TV and film. The plight of Black male actors was no different, and it was hard to visualize Black men as beautiful when usually the only parts they were given were those of the mugger, the drug dealer, the Uncle Tom, the slave.

However, that was then, back in the early 80s, and this is now, and the landscape of what is defined as Black beauty for Black women and men has changed, is changing and is heading in the right direction. The darker the berry, the sweeter the fruit. Michaela Coel, Viola Davis, Lupita Nyong'o, Gabourey Sidibe, Cynthia Erivo, Idris Elba, Omar Sy, Denzel Washington, the list is endless. Black people, POC are demanding to see themselves reflected on packaging, and brands recognize this. Money talks. Seeing Letitia Wright on the front cover of *Elle* magazine made me smile inside out.

What more do you think needs to be done to empower Black women in terms of the beauty standards set for them?

I think we have to just be in the world. Don't keep looking outside of ourselves for validation. Like we were in the past with magazines. Because it's all fake. In my opinion, beauty is an inside job. If our mothers don't recognize Black beauty within themselves, then how on earth can the young Black girl growing up in that environment recognize Black beauty within herself? It's impossible. Education will set the standard for Black women in terms of beauty, and it starts at home. Lessons Black girls learn about their Blackness and beauty at home will colour their experiences when they're out in the world trying to discover who they are and how they fit in. Our little Black girls, our daughters, our grandchildren, their Black female friends, and their friends of colour need to be told that they are beautiful when they are in our company. They need to be told that they are worthy of everything that this wide world has to offer. They need to be told their Black Lives Matter. They need to be told that they are enough. If our young Black girls see this love and acceptance demonstrated at home, within the community, our gathering spaces, churches, Mosques, Temples, etc., they will grow confident about who they are... Black, Female and BEAUTIFUL.

What advice would you give to your younger self today? Or what do you wish your younger self had known, that you know today?

You will develop a brand called Doreene Blackstock, a Black British Actress. Along the way, people will tell you that you should lower your standards and expectations because you're Black and the colour of your skin makes you unattractive. Don't believe them. People will tell you that you are unteachable because you're Black. Don't believe them. People are going to try to convince you that you're not enough. Don't believe them. And people are going to tell you things about your Black history that are bare-faced lies. Don't believe them! Learn to say "No" and mean it without apology. Demand a seat at the table, you are Black and beautiful, and you are enough.

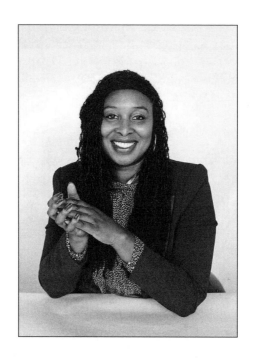

DAWN BUTLER

Dawn Butler is the elected Member of Parliament for Brent South, and served as Labour's Shadow Minister for Women and Equalities between 2017–2020.

Dawn was born and raised in Forest Gate, East London. Her parents were originally from Jamaica and she has four brothers and a sister. At a young age she worked on a market stall as well as helping out at her family's bakery store. She attended Waltham Forest College before training in IT and becoming a computer programmer/systems analyst.

She went on to work as an equality and race officer at the GMB union and became an adviser to the Mayor of London. Elected as an MP in 2005, she later became the first elected African-Caribbean woman to become a Government Minister in the UK.

Dawn was chair of the All Party Parliamentary Group on Youth Affairs and was made a member of the Children, Schools and Families select committee and Vice Chair of the Labour Party with responsibility for Youth. In 2008 she became an Assistant Whip in the Commons before her work on youth led to Dawn being appointed as the Minister for Young Citizens & Youth Engagement at the Cabinet Office by Gordon Brown.

Dawn was named the "most promising feminist under 35" by *New Statesman* magazine and was honoured as MP of the year at the 2009 Women in Public Life Awards. Dawn was awarded two Patchwork Foundation awards, having been voted People's Choice 2016 Labour MP of the Year and next receiving the Overall MP of the Year award 2017. In 2020 she was named one of the 25 most influential women in the UK by *Vogue*.

What was your go-to hairstyle as a child, and who used to do your hair?

My mum did my hair. Two cornrows either side.

Who was your hair inspiration growing up? Did you struggle to find Black hair inspiration?

Angela Davis, Bob Marley, family and friends

Who are the Black female role models in society, and how do they differ from the role models you had growing up?

With social media, there are a vast number of Black female role models now. You can find images and video tutorials online to do your hair in the comfort of your own home. I am blown away by the Black women embracing their awesomeness, I wish I'd believed and walked in my power when I was younger.

When you were young, what beauty standards did you associate with being beautiful, and how do they differ today?

The good hair language was always prevalent. Light skin and slim were the go-to beauty norms. But on saying that, I was lucky to have a father who told me I was beautiful, even if I didn't feel it. And I would strongly advise women to not waste their slim days thinking they are fat.

At what age were you made to feel like your hair was different? Tell us about that experience, what it felt like and how you navigated that?

I knew my hair was different when at school the teachers expected us to have a shower, get our hair wet and let it dry naturally. Trying to explain that we can not wash our hair and go was a mammoth feat.

What age were you when you started to make your own hair decisions, what were those decisions, and why did you choose the style you did?

At 16 or 17. I wanted to loc my hair but my parents were against it so they let me relax my hair instead.

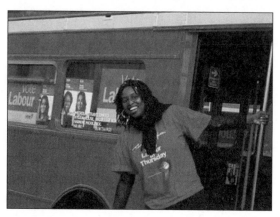

Do you have any experiences where your hair had a major effect on something in your life?

The difficulties some children with Afro hair may experience due to school policies which do not take into consideration the maintenance requirements for healthy Afro hair.

How do you wear your hair at work? Or for interviews? Has this changed over time?

My hair is in locks so I wear it down often.

What part does your hair play in your life today? What in your "hair story" helped shape that?

My hair is a symbol of self-love and appreciation of my uniqueness. And the beauty of African hair.

What do you think about how brands situate themselves in the narrative of Black hair? What more do you think could be done?

For many years straight hair was promoted on many brands which required chemical products to achieve these results. However, you will find many people have steered away from these products due to the wealth of information regarding the negative affects.

Now brands are promoting a wider range of products which include natural nourishing ingredients to care for textured hair.

What do you think of beauty products such as skin-lightening creams?

These should be banned!

Can you easily find beauty products which suit your skin tone?

There was a time when I could only find products when I went abroad. Now there are far more product ranges available here.

What do you think of the differences between the way Black men and Black women are treated in society when it comes to standards of beauty?

The colour of our skin has a direct effect on the way we are treated and viewed because of ongoing discrimination and the underrepresentaion of Black men and women in the media.

What more do you think needs to be done to empower Black women, particulary regarding hair and beauty?

First let's empower ourselves. I remember when I first got my sisterlocks done, it was like joining a club. So many women started speaking to me, saying, "Hello, I like your hair, who's your loctician?"

Having conversations with my loctician Marie, who wouldn't let me dye my hair, what I realized was how powerful it is to just acknowledge and communicate with each other. It makes a difference to just say, "Hi, the sun is out and I am in a 'let's show respect and love each other' mode."

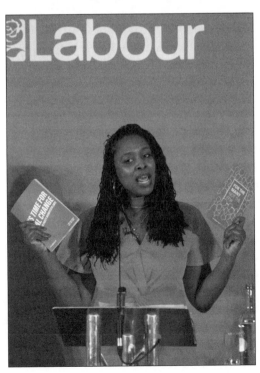

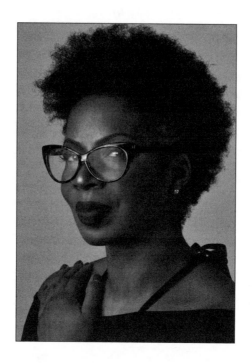

ANASTASIA CHIKEZIE

Anastasia Chikezie is the founder of the multi-award-winning hair salon, Purely Natural, one of the first natural hair salons to open in the UK in 1990. Purely Natural is attended by a host of celebrity clients such as Erykah Badu, Solange Knowles, Lena Waithe, Gina Yashere to name a few. She has created her own hair care brand, Purely Natural By Anastasia, made using organic, ethical and sustainably-sourced ingredients.

Anastasia was a regular face at Afro Hair and Beauty Show, Europe's biggest lifestyle show, where she held seminars and lectures. At trade fairs in Nigeria, she used her trichological training to diagnose and treat hair and scalp disorders, and sometimes the queue was so long she would work well into the night diagnosing and educating her clients.

Anastasia has won many awards including: Sensational Award For Best Braid 2006 & 2008, Black Woman in Business Award 2007, Sleek Hair Awards Braid Stylist 2009, Sensational Award For Best Natural Hair 2012, BE Mogul Award 2016, World Afro Day Awards, Afro Pioneer 2018, Curly Treats Festival, Excellence Stylist Award 2018.

Anastasia was creative hair stylist at Africa Fashion Week (Nigeria) where she designed and created hairstyles for 60 models, over a period of two days and was featured extensively in the media in Lagos.

Because of her extensive knowledge in natural hair she was asked to work on the expert working panel for HABIA helping to write the new NVQ qualification in Afro Hairdressing, for natural hair.

What was your go to hairstyle as a child and who used to do your hair?

Oh my gosh, my go-to hairstyle as a child? I'm of Nigerian heritage, you can tell from my Igbo surname, and I'm the oldest (Ada) of 4 daughters. When my mum came to England, she was accustomed to African threading or Isi owu – it's where they part the hair and wrap threads around the natural hair. This is a style but can be used to stretch the hair. But my mum used to leave the threads on the hair and leave the hair sticking up. So you can imagine how that looked. I didn't choose it, and I detested it because they used to call us "spider head" or "spider legs" at school. As soon as I got old enough, I used to leave home about fifteen minutes earlier than I should and rush to school and change my hairstyle. I'd take out the threads, and cornrow, plait, or twist my hair, all within fifteen minutes. Then I would leave school and rush home to rethread my hair so that when my mum got back from work, she was none the wiser. It was a mad thing, but that's how I started to do mine and my sibling's hair.

Over time, I started to get more creative and then one day, mum found out. When she realized what we were doing, she just left me to it, so at age 12, I was in charge of the rest of my sisters' hair too. There are four of us in total, and I was in charge of styling their hair. To be honest, that's where I got my wings; that's when I learnt to do styles. Natural hairstyles because we weren't allowed to relax or perm our hair. Back then, it was considered a luxury for the big people, so relaxing or perming or anything like that wasn't an option for us. One thing I remembered doing was using a fork to press hair or stretch my hair; yeah, we used to use a fork. We put it on a hot cooker ring, and when it was red hot, we ran it through the hair. Needless to say, the stench of burnt hair was a regular thing.

What do you think your mum would have done if she'd found out that you were taking your hair down when you got to school and redoing it?

We would have been reprimanded. It would have been a big deal. But later on in life, my mum told us that [she did that] because she didn't want boys to look at us. That was her reason, so she knew at that point that the hairstyle was a big deterrent in every way, shape and form. In hindsight, I guess she did what she thought she needed to do. She said, "I've got four daughters, and I don't want any boys chasing them." When I started secondary school, I first started styling my hair and looking for other styling options. When I was a lot younger, every time my parents asked me what I wanted for birthdays/ Christmas, I always used to say a doll, and that was so I could cut the hair – all my dollies had haircuts. I never played with them; my only interest was to give them a haircut. The funny thing is, for most of us hairdressers, our first haircut or attempt at a haircut was on our dollies that had European, bone straight hair.

So where did you pull your creative hair inspirations from?

I think it came naturally; it's in my DNA. My mum was into clothes and fashion and 50 or so years ago attended the famous London College of Fashion. She was a creative, and [she] inspired me.

Did you ever look for inspiration from anywhere else? When you were young, did you have anyone on TV that you looked at for example?

Not at all. Now we have social media, so there are high profile Black celebrities which we can look up to, but back then, I don't recall any. I used to read a

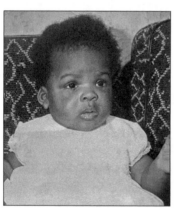

mag called *Mandy* which was a typically white magazine. All the characters in there were white with bone straight hair. This was very typical of TV back then. I was fostered. I don't really like to talk about this, but a white family fostered me for the first six years of my life, and my hair wasn't combed or groomed. It wasn't even touched. I think they used to just wash it and go daily. You can't wash and go 4C hair, without product as you know, but they would just wash my hair and leave it to air dry, so my hair was just a matted mess. All the other children fostered to the same family were all white, and their hair was the complete opposite to mine, so I had no inspiration at a very young age. In fact, quite the opposite. But I don't recall hating my hair or having any issues with the way I looked. They always made me feel part of the family. I had no concerns about how I looked or the fact I was different. But obviously, as I got older, we had Lauryn Hill. She inspired many. I tried to model myself off her and locked my hair for the first time. Thirty-odd years ago, I opened the first natural hair salon.

Was there a time when you were made to feel that your hair was different?

Not that I recall. The only thing that frightened me was when I saw images of myself when I got older with my matted hair. I knew at that point that my foster parents didn't know how to care for my hair, but I don't recall any standout situation that I felt affected me negatively – unless I've blocked it out. Selective memory can be a wonderful thing at times.

Before you opened Purely Natural, did you ever have a job role that made you wear your hair a certain way or was there a defining moment when you were made to feel that you needed to fit into the environment?

No. To be honest, for most of my life, I've worked for myself. I only had one job in a fast food takeaway in Piccadilly Circus, but it wasn't a job where I had to change my hairstyle. A defining moment was when I met a young man I married and had three children with him, and we both embarked on a fully vegan lifestyle. I decided to cut my hair during that time. I went down to a really low cut with a fade, and I wore my hair like that for years.

Another defining moment was when I went back to university as a mature student to study Psychology and Law. I remember going in with my natural fade. As my hair started to grow out, I started to experiment with twists and colours. People used to stop me and were like, "Who did your hair?" It was crazy; every day, someone would approach me. I told them that I did my hair, and they would ask if I could do theirs. So, I started inviting clients to my home, but my husband wasn't happy because the kids were quite young and having strangers come in and out of our home wasn't ideal. So he had a small barbershop, and he said he'd prefer it if I did the clients in the shop. In the evenings and during the summer and Easter holidays, I was in the salon. My clientele grew, and so did my staff – it was like an overnight thing. By the time I graduated, I had a full team, and it just made sense to develop that. Then a couple of years later, I went back to college and got my NVQ in Hairdressing and then, I went on to do Trichology and Cosmetology.

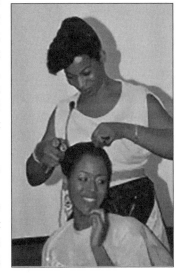

Did you train your staff, or did they come to you, trained?

Oh, I trained them! At the time, I used to travel a lot, so I'd go to America to see what they were doing up there, pick up magazines and then have a day in the salon where I'd say,

OK, I've seen this on TV, let's see how we can replicate it. So, when Alicia Keys came with her style, cornrows and one over the ear, we practised it. As soon as I saw it somewhere, I'd bring the style into the salon, and I'd practise with the girls. From the locks to the braiding. They had to have a minimum skill which was to be able to plait, but everything else I trained them in. And when I went to America I used to bring back a whole load of extensions, because back then, America was a lot more forward than we were in terms of natural hair so they had all the extensions before we did. I'd go there, pick up extensions, hair nets and loads of little things that I hadn't seen before and bring them and get the staff to practise on each other until we got it right, so by the time we were ready to open we had Alicia Keys' hairstyle down to a tee, we had Lauryn Hill's hairstyle down to a tee, we had Whitney Houston's down to a tee.

What did you see other Black people sporting at the time you were learning these new American styles?

They were all doing relaxers and curly perms! That was the big thing in the seventies and eighties. People used to think we were crazy and say, "Why don't you do relaxers? You're missing a big market there!" I used to get pulled up all the time for not wanting to deal with chemicals. But for us, it wasn't just the hair, it was our whole liberty. We were using natural organic haircare and skincare with no chemicals, and all our treatments were natural and organic. Even when my kids went to school, their packed lunch used to have vegan milk. But we did get a lot of opposition from the community. And now everyone's doing it.

And now everyone's doing it. What do you think about that?

It's given me the title 'pioneer' now, which I really appreciate. Even though

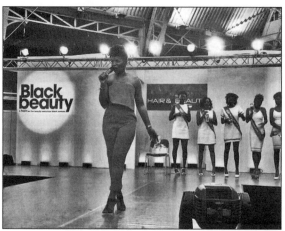

that wasn't my intention at the time, it was just me, and I wasn't making a statement; it was just my liberty. We're born with natural hair, and it's our birthright. We're proud of our hair and the way we look in our natural state. So, I wasn't concerned, but I know that there were concerns over natural hair from others. We'd have clients come in concerned over their hair because they had a job interview or had to go work in the corporate world. Or a client would want natural styles, but they didn't want anything too radical, dimming their Blackness. I know back then, there was an agenda, and many people had bad experiences because of that. I know times are changing but back then, it was a major issue, so we'd have clients qualifying in the legal profession as a barrister, and they'd come in after their first interview, and they'd be concerned over how they would be perceived with their locks, and they'd come to cut them off.

Over the years, I've noticed how our clientele has changed. Back then, our clientele were middle-aged women who had done the relaxer and lost hair or done the curly perm, wigs, lost hair and came full circle. They were going through menopause or were experiencing hair loss, and they just came to me because they were concerned and didn't know what to do next. So, it was a last resort to go natural back then. They would come in and say, "I'm scared about going natural. I don't know what my hair looks like. I don't know how to handle it." What the hell?! Can you imagine? Now our clients are as young as 11, and they're coming in and saying they want their hair parted into four, twisted, blow-dried. Children as young as 11 say that they want shampoo one week and then a co wash the following week, and that they don't want heat on their hair and know when it's time for a trim. I think another wind of change has come. We had the older generation, and then we had an era when it was mostly younger women. Now fifty per cent of my clients are young guys because, to an extent, women are self-sufficient. They know how to fling in a couple of cornrows if need be, but guys don't, so there is a new wind now.

Back then, the natural hair movement was always associated with looking dowdy, in my opinion. I used to come in with my natural hair, red lipstick, and heels, but back then, women who wore their natural hair always looked dowdy. So, when I started seeing all these young sisters out there with natural hair and looking sexy with it, I was like, "Yes! It's about time!" Seeing powerful, sexy Black women with a head full of natural hair – it took long enough. This isn't a political statement. This is our hair, our birthright. We can still wear our tight jeans and our mini-skirts and heels and rock that natural hair as that wasn't happening back then. I'm glad things have done a 360-degree turn, and now wearing our hair in its natural state is not frowned upon.

Did you notice any more diversity with Black women's hair in America?

Yeh definitely. At the time, America definitely used to lead the way. In America, there was a lot more variety in terms of styling, even the extensions.

You could find natural-looking hair extensions back then in America when you couldn't get them here. Just walking around over there, you'd see the odd person sporting their natural hairstyle – more so than in England. America provided a lot of inspiration. So, if you were going to America and picking up styles, you'd always be ahead because they were ahead.

What do you think of the differences in the ways that Black men and Black women are treated when it comes to their hair?

I used to find that the way I wore my hair determined what kind of guys would approach me. So, when I wore long braids down my back, I'd get younger men. When I wore locks, I got many Rastafarians, hailing me with "Sister, respect, respect," and when I had my hair short, people automatically assumed I was a lesbian. If I was wearing my hair in an Afro, apparently, I was making a political statement. It's crazy how the way we wear our hair affects how people perceive us. It's big. It's not just a small perception; they look at us and prejudge us based on the way we wore our hair. Oh, and getting male attention with twisted hair was down to a minimum. Unfortunately, the way a man perceives us, does to a certain extent, dictate the kind of hairstyles we choose. I don't know if that applies across the board, but I know specifically when it comes to Black hair, people think that they can get a sense of us based on how we wear our hair. For me, all I care about is healthy hair, no matter what you do with it. It hurts when clients come in, and they've been wearing weave for the longest time, and their hair is not healthy underneath. Out of sight should not be out of mind. Put that wig or that weave back on if you want, but remember alopecia is a real thing, so be mindful and give yourself a break now and again. But when women come in and say they don't want to see their hair, they do not like their hair, so they do back-to-back weaves, I have a major problem with that. That is crazy to me. Education is key. But I think we're getting there. I see it happening, and I think we are getting to the point where we can wear our natural hair without feeling like we're being stigmatized or perceived in any way because we're choosing to wear our hair in its natural state.

What more do you think needs to be done to empower Black women?

There's a lot of education that needs to be done. More social media groups are being formed: love your hair and love the skin you're in, but we need to see many more dark-skinned sisters with 4C hair in the media; they need to be showcased. We need to do education in schools concerning basic haircare. Hair is part of us. They do a lot of courses on nutrition in school, but I think hair needs to be tied into that in some way. Self-love and acceptance are really important, especially in the formative years. But we're getting there – slowly.

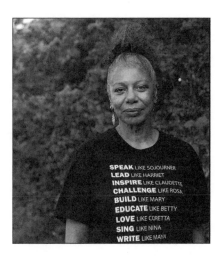

STELLA DADZIE

Stella Dadzie is a writer and historian best known for her co-authorship of *The Heart of the Race: Black Women's Lives in Britain* which won the 1985 Martin Luther King Award for Literature. She is a founder member of OWAAD (Organisation of Women of African and Asian Descent), and was recently described as one of the "grandmothers" of Black Feminism in the UK. Her career as a teacher, writer, artist and education activist spans over 40 years. She is well known within the UK for her contribution to tackling youth racism and working with racist perpetrators, and is a key contributor to the development of anti-racist strategies with schools, colleges and youth services. She has run workshops, spoken at many international conferences and was a guest Lecturer at Havard University in 2018.

She appeared in *And Still I Rise,* a documentary exploring the social and historical origins of stereotypes of African women, and was a guest of Germaine Greer on her BBC2 discussion programme, *The Last Word.*

What was your go-to hairstyle as a child, and who used to do your hair?

My (white) mother styled my hair in large curls the size of pennies when I was a baby, but once the kink appeared, she despaired, she didn't know what to do with it. I have an early memory of the woman who used to look after me after school tearing a comb through my tangles and slapping me for crying because she was literally tearing it out at the roots. She obviously thought she could 'tame' my hair, something which my mother was clearly failing to do. I would have been about four years old at the time. As I grew older, my mother's solution was to tell me to cover my hair with a headscarf. To her it was an embarrassment, something to be hidden from view. This was the 1950s, when a white woman with a 'coloured' child was often assumed to be a prostitute or a 'loose' woman. Some people spat at her in the street. So to my mother, my frizzy hair was evidence of her shame.

Who was your hair inspiration growing up? Did you struggle to find Black hair inspiration?

I didn't have any hair inspiration as a young child, not that I can remember. It was only when I was introduced to my (Ghanaian) father's side of the family that I began to see Black women with straightened hair. For my 13th birthday, my step-mum, who in my eyes was the height of sophistication, paid for me to have my hair straightened at Raymond's of Knightsbridge, the posh, white hairdressing salon she frequented when she visited London. I came out with sleek, straight hair which I loved, but no one explained to me that to keep it straight, I would need to put it in rollers whenever I washed it or got it wet. I was devastated when it 'reverted' the first time I washed my hair. I rang my step-mum in tears, and told her it hadn't worked. She arranged for me to go back to the hairdresser who did it again. As a result, the hair broke all over the top of my head. I was left with long hair at the sides and a half inch of hair growth on top, and was so embarrassed, I remember I wore a hair-piece to try to cover it up. I was the only Black girl in my school, and my hair was already an embarrassment, so I was mortified.

Who are the Black female role models in society, and how do they differ from the role models you had growing up?

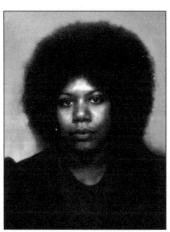

Women like Tracy Chapman and Erykah Badu are very different to the icons I grew up with. My role models, if you can call them that, were singers like Shirley Bassey and Millie Small, both of whom wore their hair straight. In fact, looking at a picture of her, I think Millie wore a wig. In those days, you wouldn't have stood a chance in show-business if you'd appeared on stage with natural hair. Later, when Motown singers began to appear on *Top of the Pops*, we would see women like Diana Ross & the Supremes. Again, they always wore wigs or had their hair relaxed.

When you were young, what beauty standards did you associate with being beautiful, and how do they differ today?

To a little girl of mixed race growing up in the 50s and 60s, beauty was associated with long, sleek hair, ideally blonde, invariably European. Marilyn Monroe comes to mind, and women like Brigitte Bardot, Raquel Welch and Elizabeth Taylor. There simply were no Black women to emulate or look up to. Black women were invisible in the movies and on TV, and if they ever did feature, they were maids, cleaners or prostitutes. Black women were rarely given enviable roles until Civil Rights, when things began to change. After that, there was a spate of 'blaxploitation' movies, like *Cleopatra Jones* and *Shaft*, and the women often sported Afros. For my generation, that was probably the first time we had ever seen Black women depicted as glamorous or sexually attractive.

At what age were you made to feel like your hair was different? Tell us about that experience, what it felt like and how you navigated that?

I was aware that my hair was different from a very early age, probably from around four years old.

What age were you when you started to make your own hair decisions, what were those decisions, and why did you choose the style you did?

When I was 19 or 20, I started wearing my hair in a large Afro. I was inspired by Angela Davis and the messages coming from the Black Power movement at the time – messages like 'Say it loud, I'm Black and I'm proud' and 'to be young, gifted and Black is where it's at' which were popular songs coming from America. Wearing an Afro was a statement to the world, a declaration that young Black women like myself were no longer prepared to buy into the idea that our hair was something to be ashamed of.

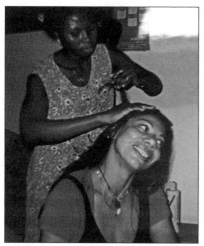

After that, for many years I wore my hair in plaits – usually with extensions. I'd go home to Ghana and head for Nima, which is a poor area in Accra with countless hairdressers who would plait your hair for a pittance. I remember one woman asking me how big I wanted my plaits. I replied "kakraba, kakraba'. In Fante, if you repeat a word, it's a way of turning the word into a superlative, so I was unwittingly telling her to do them really small. When I got home, my auntie took one look at me and said 'those plaits are criminal!' They were tiny! Of course, the problem arose when I got back to the UK and eventually had to take them out. It would tear the hair out at the roots. A lot of Black women suffered from traction alopecia because of all the plaiting. The weight of the extensions and the fact that they were attached to just a few strands of hair took a serious toll.

Do you have any experiences where your hair had a major effect on something in your life?

When I began going through my menopause, my hair got really thin at the front. It got so bad, I went to a hair clinic and was prescribed Minoxidil. It was all hard-sell – no attempt to analyse the cause of the hair loss or suggest alternative ways to treat it. I was told to put the cream they'd prescribed on my hair last thing at night. It transferred to my pillow, and I soon noticed a fine down growing across my cheeks. I also began to feel really unwell. I went back to the clinic and complained. I'd discovered that the recommended dosage was 5% yet they had prescribed 12.5%, which my doctor was horrified about, because it was an unlicensed product. I remember the woman I spoke with at the clinic telling me "Oh, we give all the Black girls 12.5%", yet they had never once asked me my ethnicity. I had to have my hair analysed by a trichologist, who discovered that although I had my father's hair colour and texture, I had inherited my mother's fine hair structure. It also transpired that my hair loss was caused by my menopause, not traction alopecia as I had been told, so the follicles were actually dead. I took the Hair Clinic to court and eventually won my case, but it was a traumatic experience.

What part does your hair play in your life today? What in your 'hair story' helped shape that?

My hair is completely natural – I can't remember the last time I did anything drastic to it. I simply wash it, condition my scalp and tie it back so it's out of my face. I prefer my hair to look a bit natty, but if I go to the hairdressers she always tongs it so it looks sleek and European. As soon as I get home, I tie it back and wet it so it reverts to its natural curl. My hairdresser would have a fit if she knew! Until last year I used to darken my roots but once lockdown kicked in I decided to let it go grey. I couldn't go out to buy hair colour, so why bother? I'm getting used to my grey hair now – and I'm at peace with it.

Now I'm older, my hair doesn't play a big part it my life. As long as it's presentable, I forget about it. I should probably cut it short, but I'm used to the way it looks, so why risk changing it?

What do you think about how brands situate themselves in the narrative of Black hair? What more do you think could be done?

If you go into any shop selling Black hair products, there are aisles and aisles of hair products, all promising to do the impossible. Black women spend a fortune on trying to 'tame' our hair, it's a multimillion dollar industry with relaxers for children that contain dangerous chemicals, curl custards, all kinds of foolishness. These days, more and more Black women have begun to challenge the need for these products. But if you browse the Black hair magazines in the hairdressers, it's the same old story – endless advertisements for wigs, extensions and relaxers. You do see more Afrocentric styles featured these days, but we have a way to go before we truly rid ourselves of all those centuries of conditioning, telling us to aspire to a European standard of hair beauty.

What do you think of the differences between the way Black men and Black women are treated in society when it comes to standards of beauty?

We've all been through the same process, it's just that men are less pressured than women, or at least they used to be. Men are more likely to wear their hair short, but they are still subjected to the same hard-sell when it comes to hair products. I think Black men have had a similar journey, it's just less discussed. The 'brothers' stopped using curly-perms and started wearing Afros just like we did back in the 70s. Black men seem more and more fetishized these days, but they have had to contend with the same marketing messages, the same mental colonization and the same self-hatred.

What more do you think needs to be done to empower Black women, particularly regarding hair and beauty?

I think it's about having more positive role models – Black women who are proud of who they are and how they look, who don't need to emulate whiteness in order to feel beautiful. There should certainly be a ban on advertising skin bleaching creams and hair relaxers for children.

What advice would you give to your younger self today? Or, what do you wish your younger self had known, that you know today?

To recognize my own beauty.

Anything else you'd like to add?

Only that these questions have made me focus on my 'hair journey' in a way I've never really done before. They've certainly helped me to acknowledge how much trauma my hair has caused me at different times in my life!

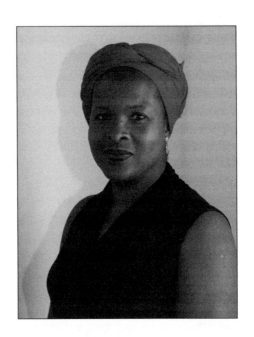

SOKARI DOUGLAS CAMP

Sokari Douglas Camp CBE was born in Buguma, Rivers State, Nigeria. She studied fine art at Central School of Art and Design and at the Royal College of Art. Sokari has represented Britain and Nigeria in national exhibitions and has had more than 40 solo shows worldwide, in venues such as National Museum of African Art, Smithsonian Institute 1988–89, the Museum of Mankind, London 1994–5. Her public artworks include *Battle Bus: Living Memorial for Ken Saro-Wiwa* (2006), a full-scale replica of a Nigerian steel bus, which stands as a monument to the late Niger Delta activist and writer. *'All the World is Now Richer'*, a memorial to commemorate the abolition of slavery was exhibited in The House of Commons 2012 and St Paul's Cathedral 2014.

Working with steel is very physical, and she used to joke that this was a way of keeping warm in the UK, but, she enjoys the repetition of welding cutting and bending metal into shape. In 2003 Sokari was shortlisted for the Trafalgar Square Fourth Plinth. Her work is in permanent collections at The Smithsonian Museum, Washington, D.C., Setagaya Museum, Tokyo and the British Museum, London. In 2005 she was awarded a CBE in recognition of her services to art.

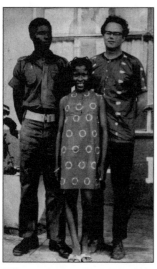

What was your go-to hairstyle as a child, and who used to do your hair?

Cornrows and thread styles.

Who was your hair inspiration growing up? Did you struggle to find Black hair inspiration?

No real struggles with hair; inspiration from my family in Nigeria and from Afros in the 70s in the US.

Who are the Black female role models in society, and how do they differ from the role models you had growing up?

Angela Davis, Dianne Abbott. Growing up my mother and sister.

When you were young, what beauty standards did you associate with being beautiful, and how do they differ today?

When I was young, my main beauty standard was my sister; her beauty was close to being ugly to some. But she was considered fascinating, a real beauty.

Can you remember when you were first made to feel like your hair was different? Tell us about that experience, what it felt like and how you navigated that?

A boy wanted a 'lock 'of my hair. White friends usually needed scissors to cut a lock. I broke a tuft from my Afro… that has always stuck with me because my Afro is like cotton while white hair is a little tougher, maybe like silk.

What age were you when you started to make your own hair decisions, what were those decisions, and why did you choose the style you did?

I was eight when I started making hair decisions and when in Nigeria, I chose what was in fashion, styles with string or cornrows.

What part does your hair play in your life today? What in your "hair story" helped shaped that?

My hair is thinning and balding in my sixties and I think this is a part of the menopause that was never explained to me.

What do you think about how brands situate themselves in the narrative of Black hair? What more do you think could be done?

I think I am part of a generation that did not know much about hair products. We went with what we were given in salons and on the street, at hair stalls…

Afro brand shops are crazy. I still do not know what to pick, except things with argan oil, shea butter or olive oil.

Do you think there is a difference in the way Black men and Black women are treated in society when it comes to standards of beauty?

In white societies yes. In African societies, European wigs are now popular with women which is very odd.

What more do you think needs to be done to empower Black women, particularly regarding hair and beauty?

We need the support of our men; wigs are not ok, and we need to touch our own hair in public and in the media.

What advice would you give to your younger self today? Or what do you wish your younger self had known, that you know today?

Love your hair while you have it, because it is beautiful.

Anything else you want to say?

There should be a video of Black hair being touched... not just how to manage our hair with some product, just general appreciation of our hair. White hair is constantly being flicked, touched, swept back, whirled around. When it comes to Black hair there is only: "Do not touch." Wet Black hair with water glistening on it is a sight to behold...(hahaha) So textured and complicated it is wonderful.

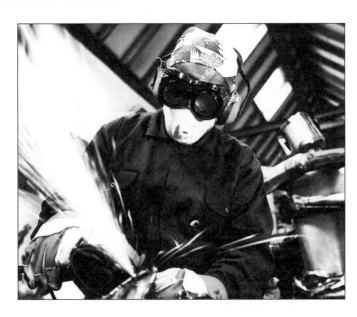

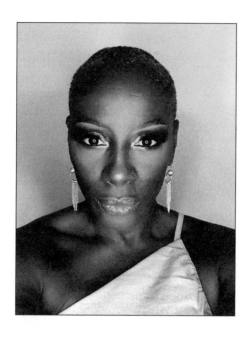

STEPHANIE DOUGLAS OLY

Stephanie is an 8 times British Athletics Champion who competed in the 100m at two Olympic Games (1992 and 1996). She also represented Team GB at several World Championships (1991, 1995, 1999) and is a European (1990) and Commonwealth (1990, 1994) relay medalist and an individual finalist. She is still amongst the UK's all-time fastest sprinters.

Since retiring from athletics, Stephanie has continued to support British athletics as a sprint coach for the Great Britain athletics team at the 2007 World University Games and has coached teenage athletes, to achieve their full potential, for Watford Athletics Club.

Stephanie is a fully qualified Soft Tissue Therapist providing a range of sports and remedial massage techniques to prevent and treat injuries, optimising the healing process. To add to these skills, she is studying for a Science degree in Sport and Exercise Rehabilitation.

Stephanie has one daughter called Jorja. They both competed in a series of challenges whilst appearing on series 2 of CBBC's singing talent show, *Got What It Takes?*, winning the competition and the opportunity for Jorja to perform on the Main Stage at the 2017 Radio 1's Big Weekend.

What was your go-to hairstyle as a child, and who used to do your hair?

My go-to hairstyle was whatever my mum did to my hair. Options were very limited. I remember we had a hot comb which had to go on the stove; relaxer kits were becoming available, and my mum would put our hair in Chiney Bumps (Bantu knots) on Sunday evenings to make it reasonably manageable throughout the school week. I recall the experience of sitting between my mum's legs and getting chopped with the comb every time I didn't sit still or turned my head to avoid the pain – fond memories indeed. For school, my hair was left out or put in one or two bunches. Around age nine, my mum decided to relax my hair which ended disastrously as it all fell out, and when I went to school I had to endure endless taunting.

Who was your hair inspiration growing up? Did you struggle to find Black hair inspiration?

Growing up in the 70s, I didn't come into contact with many Black women around Manchester apart from my auntie and my mum. There were not many Black children and no Black teachers in school. We had three channels on TV that did not offer many programmes featuring Black women. My mum wore her hair natural or permed until she got married (when I was 12), and then she wore beautiful braids. When the curly perm was fashionable in the 80s, I asked for that style which made my hair slightly softer and more manageable.

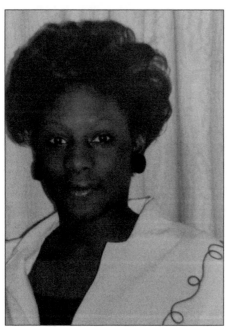

Who are the Black female role models in society, and how do they differ from the role models you had growing up?

Throughout my teens, twenties and thirties, I used to change my hairstyle every week whether it was my own hair, putting a wig on, adding some extensions or Ghana braids. I tried everything and looked at the different styles of other women. I loved Sade's and Whitney Houston's styles. Whitney fascinated me with a different hairstyle in each of her music videos. Now it's so different, especially with social media. I see Black female role models in all aspects of life.

I am particularly inspired by Serena Williams for the way she has stayed at the top of her industry for so many years. I also gain inspiration from women who look like me – dark and bald – who embrace their skin and hairstyle choice.

When you were young, what beauty standards did you associate with being beautiful, and how do they differ today?

When I was young, I associated the typical "blonde hair and blue eyes" with being beautiful and my female idol was Debbie Harry. As I've aged, I know that beauty comes from within, although a little make-up can enhance your features. As long as you feel good in yourself, nobody should be able to dull that shine. Nowadays, I like looking at dark-skinned women, who I associate with, and I appreciate their beauty.

At what age were you made to feel that your hair was different? Tell us about that experience, what it felt like and how you navigated that?

I always knew my hair was different, since I grew up and lived in predominantly white areas, therefore attending predominantly white schools. The episode where my mum decided to relax my hair, leaving the relaxer on too long, consequently resulted in taunts of "boy" and "picky head" from my peers. I just had to hold out until my hair grew back which took quite a while. The dreaded British weather was also a nightmare to navigate. As soon as any rain or too much sun hit, the shrinkage was unbearable and my "friends" or even strangers would come up and put their hands in my hair.

What age were you when you started to make your own hair decisions, what were those decisions, and why did you choose the style you did?

It was probably my early teens because, as an athlete, I needed a style that was easy to manage whilst training and competing. Having to run in the rain would affect the chemicals in the curly perm so I would carry my bottle of curl activator around. Once I moved down to London around the age of 19, I started mixing with more Black people and had easy access to Black hair salons and shops. I just went crazy with my hairstyles. My hairdresser became a close friend. When looking back through old photographs and videos from athletics days, I sometimes question my hairstyle decisions!

Do you have any experiences where your hair had a major effect on something in your life?

I do what I want with my hair. As long as I like it, no one can say anything that will make me change it. I recall an incident after I made the decision to shave my head. I had just started dating a guy and I told him of my pending baldness. He said he would see how he felt once I had done it. He couldn't handle the subsequent change and we parted ways shortly after. I also do get annoyed when shop assistants, waiters, or customer-facing staff assume that I am a man and call me "Sir!"

How do you wear your hair at work? Or for interviews? Has this changed over time?

I've been bald since 2017 so I don't really worry about my hair now. Sometimes I shave it clean and sometimes I have a little growth. It still requires maintenance especially when I want the clean-shaven look. Pre-bald, I changed my style so often, my colleagues sometimes didn't recognize me!

What part does your hair play in your life today? What in your "hair story" helped shape that?

My lack of hair plays a major role in my life. I've done so much to my hair over my five decades and I am happy with the style I've been wearing for the past four years. I have a blank canvas and can choose to sport a long, curly, straight style or any other style at any time. As I am postmenopausal, the thought of having hair on my head is not appealing especially when I am experiencing a hot flush.

What do you think about how brands situate themselves in the narrative of Black hair? What more do you think could be done?

I feel that the brands and the shops which are selling their products are ripping us off. They're too expensive; it costs a fortune to maintain Black or mixed hair and I'm sure it doesn't need to be that price. It can be so difficult finding the right combination of products to feed our hair, although I don't have that problem anymore, but my daughter does. It would be great to have more Black-owned hair brands/shops who are educated and understand what ingredients are needed to maintain the different types of Black hair.

What do you think of beauty products such as skin-lightening creams?

I've never really understood the desire to lighten the skin. I am happy with the colour of my skin and I accept the flaws. I don't wear make-up on a daily basis and I prefer my skin to be as dark as possible, enjoying the sun when it's here.

Can you easily find beauty products which suit your skin tone?

Growing up and into my twenties the main product I used was eyeliner. I never wore full make-up, especially foundation as I found it difficult to find the right shade. There were brands like Fashion Fair back then but I only used their lipsticks for special occasions. With my full-time athletics training, it wasn't worth wearing make-up. It's gotten much easier to find my colour as most brands are making an effort to support all skin tones. I am always on the look-out for companies with make-up targeting the dark-skinned woman.

What do you think of the differences between the way Black men and Black women are treated in society when it comes to standards of beauty?

I think there is a problem with colourism in the Black community and society in general, whereby the darker-skinned Black women get the raw deal, whereas, with Black men, any shade goes.

What more do you think needs to be done to empower Black women, particularly regarding hair and beauty?

We need to challenge and respond to society whenever a Black woman is portrayed as aggressive when she stands up for herself. To keep on embracing our natural styles so that they become "a norm". I think things are going in the right direction with many influential Black women publicly highlighting these issues. It is also important to educate our daughters and sons that however they want to wear their hair, they need to feel beautiful from the inside and that will come through on the outside.

What advice would you give to your younger self today? Or, what do you wish your younger self had known, that you know today?

I would have pulled people up for putting their hands in my hair to let them know that it's not acceptable. I was ridiculed at school for having a big bottom, bigger lips and dark skin which affected my self-esteem – I needed someone to tell me that one day it would be all the rage so I could have enjoyed my natural gifts!

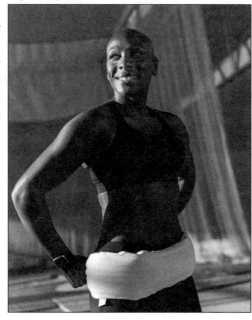

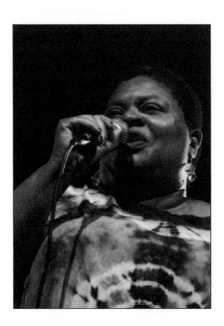

DEITRA FARR

Deitra Farr is considered one of Chicago's top vocalists, who has been nominated for Traditional Female Blues Artist of the year by the W.C. Handy Awards, Female Blues Artist of the year by the Living Blues Critics Awards, the British Blues Connection Awards, and the Les Trophées France Blues Awards. In 2015, she was inducted into the Chicago Blues Hall of Fame and in 2016 the National Southern Soul Foundation gave Deitra The Most Popular Blues Artist Award. Deitra is also the recipient of the 2017 Jus' Blues Music Foundation's Koko Taylor Queen of the Blues Award.

This Chicago native began her career in 1975, singing with local soul bands, before starting her blues career in the early 1980s. When Deitra was 18 years old, she recorded the lead vocals on Mill Street Depo's record 'You Won't Support Me'. That record was a Cashbox Top 100 R&B hit in 1976. Over 30 years later, that recording has been re-released and is popular again worldwide. She began her blues career working at the major Chicago blues clubs, then toured the US and Canada with the Sam Lay Blues Band. From 1993 to 1996, Deitra was also the lead singer with Mississippi Heat, before resuming her solo career in 1997. She has since toured Europe and the US with numerous bands including the all-star blues group Chicago Wind and has performed at the Chicago Blues Festival among many others.

From 2006–2010 Deitra toured with The Women of Chicago Blues project alongside Zora Young and Grana Louise. She is also a published writer, poet, songwriter, and painter. A graduate of Columbia College (Bachelor of Arts in Journalism), Deitra has recorded many of her own compositions and has written articles for the *Chicago Daily Defender, The Chicago Blues Annual,* and the Italian blues magazine *il Blues.* Currently she has a column "Artist to Artist" in *Living Blues* Magazine.

The Italian newspaper, the *Pistoia La Nationale,* proclaimed Deitra Farr "Regina del Blues".

What was your go-to hairstyle as a child, and who used to do your hair?

I'm a child of the 50s, 60s and 70s. My original hair was and is kinky and also called coarse. At a young age, my mother would have my hair pressed with a straightening comb/hot comb and a curling iron. Straight hair was considered good hair. My maternal grandmother used to tell me my mother messed up my "good hair", but she never told me how it was done. Maybe when I was a baby my hair was different. The worse part of getting my hair pressed was getting my ears burnt accidentally by the straightening comb. So little Black girls in America are taught quite young that something is wrong with them. Something is wrong with their hair. Little Black boys are allowed to keep their hair natural.

Who was your hair inspiration growing up? Did you struggle to find Black hair inspiration?

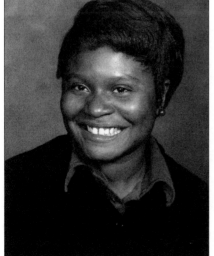

I had no hair inspiration as a child. In the mid-1960s and beyond, Black women started to allow their hair to go natural. My mother, my aunts and myself went natural. Most of the years since then I've remained natural. I got briefly bored in high school in the 1970s and got a permanent and dyed my hair auburn. Then another period around 1979 I got another permanent. Both times I made those changes for a brief time. I am not comfortable with straight hair.

Who are the Black female role models in society, and how do they differ from the role models you had growing up?

I would say entertainers are the biggest role models in society. We see them on television and in the media. When I was young we had women like Diana Ross, Diahann Carroll and Cicely Tyson to look up to. I remember back in the day, Black women entertainers often wore wigs, so they could change their looks often. I've been an entertainer for 45 years and my hair has remained natural most of the time.

When you were young, what beauty standards did you associate with being beautiful, and how do they differ today?

When I was young I always thought Black was beautiful. I always was attracted to uniqueness. I loved it that Black people have a wide range of skin colors. I loved to see a woman stand out from the crowd. I remember seeing Billie Holiday on an album cover when I was young. Her look made me want to listen to the album. To me she had a unique style. I grew up in a world that didn't appreciate dark skin very much. I remember in elementary school very dark girls would be made fun of. I thought their dark skin was beautiful. Both of my grandmothers spoke of good hair and bad hair. I found that talk irritating. Black kinky hair, of course, was the bad hair. When my mother died she had natural hair. Her mother, my grandmother insisted that they straighten her hair for the funeral. I was furious. My grandmother said, "She looked better with straight hair."

At what age were you made to feel like your hair was different? Tell us about that experience, what it felt like and how you navigated that?

I grew up on the southside of Chicago in a Black community, so most of us pretty much had the same kind of hair.

What age were you when you started to make your own hair decisions, what were those decisions, and why did you choose the style you did?

I was allowed to change my hair as a teenager, but most of the time it stayed natural.

Do you have any experiences where your hair had a major effect on something in your life?

My natural hair got me fired from a band I was singing with in the mid 1970s. The band leader wanted me to straighten my hair, because he said I looked too militant. I was not about to let a man decide how I wore my hair. In the 1970s I'd changed my hair a few times, but it was my decision. How I wear my hair will always be my decision.

What part does your hair play in your life today? What in your "hair story" helped shape that?

I am near my 64th year now and everybody knows and accepts my hair as is.

What do you think about how brands situate themselves in the narrative of Black hair? What more do you think could be done?

There are plenty of products these days to cover every type of Black hair. The varieties are vast.

What do you think of the differences between the way Black men and Black women are treated in society when it comes to standards of beauty?

Black men are not judged as harshly over their appearance, as Black women are. A man can wear the same suit every day for a year and most people would not even notice. I think we can all agree a woman could not get away with that.

What more do you think needs to be done to empower Black women, particularly regarding hair and beauty?

A woman just needs to love herself. Little Black girls should be taught they are beautiful and worthy. Then they can become women who love themselves.

What advice would you give to your younger self today? Or, what do you wish your younger self had known, that you know today?

I would tell myself I am worthy, because I did not get that message when I was young. It took me a lot of time and years to learn that I was worthy. Having self-worth is everything.

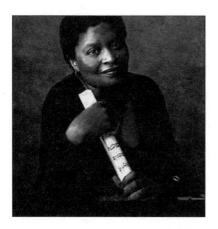

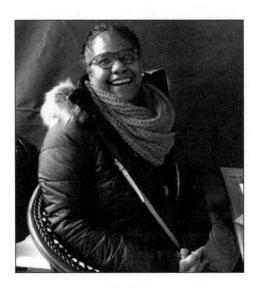

RACHEL FLEMING-CAMPBELL

Rachel Fleming-Campbell has been an attorney at Law since 1996 and a solicitor since 2004. She is qualified to practise law in two different jurisdictions: New York and England. As a litigator her speciality is Industrial Diseases and she has conducted and won several high profile cases. But she considers her greatest success in life is being a mother and raising her children.

What was your go-to her style as a child and who used to do your hair?

Three plaits, one in the front, two in the back. I had very thick hair. My mom would try to comb my hair once a week so she used to try to put me on her lap and once I actually bit her. She was so cross that she took a pair of scissors and she just cut off all my hair. I wore a hat for a very long time after that. It must have been about five or six months. My mom still has the scar in her side from where I bit her. She always talks about it.

It was not a very good experience so I've been going to the hairdressers from a very early age. According to my mom, I was born with an exceptional amount of hair on my head, very thick; she was not impressed.

Who was your hair inspiration growing up?

Actually, I didn't have anyone. I was born in London, but I grew up in Grenada. There was no such thing as hair inspiration or anything like that, but I had

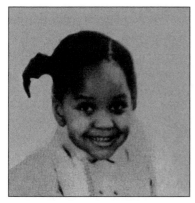

a friend who would change my hairstyle at school, so I could fit in but as I went home for lunch I would have to change my hairstyle like three, four times a day to make sure that I had the same style as my grandmother had given me in the morning.

Often she would do funny styles – it would be what I called horns – one sticking out here and one sticking out there and one on the back, as opposed to what my friends had – these really nice cornrows.

Who were your Black female role models growing up?

My grandmother, my mother and my teacher, Ms. Williams. I was dyslexic, and Ms. Williams basically taught me to read out loud. My grandmother told me that I was gifted and that I could do whatever I wanted. My mom told me that, "No is never an answer", so I never looked at those people on television, because they were not people I could touch. My grandmother was an entrepreneur, she ran her own business and my mom was a single mom. Still, we travelled the world and so I never believed that there were any barriers that I couldn't overcome. They were fantastic.

At what age were you made to feel like your hair was different? Tell us about that experience, what it felt like and how you navigated that?

I never realized my hair was different until I was at university. People would say, "Is this your hair?" And then their hands would be on my head and I hated it. Because of that, I started to braid my hair. Once I went to a trichologist and he examined my scalp and he said, "Do you realize how many hairs you have growing out of your follicles? I've never seen anything like it."

How old were you when you started to make your own hair decisions?

I basically have three people I trust to do my hair. I've been going to the same hairdresser since 1996 in London. I've had the same hairdresser in New York since 1991 and when I go to Grenada, I go to the same hairdresser. I don't do much with my hair and I think that's the reason why my hair has been in the same condition. Apart from putting in a relaxer, which I stopped in 2015, and dying it, because I am now gray, I haven't done much with my hair, so I don't experiment.

When you go to work, do you have a special hairdo?

Due to lockdown in this country, we haven't really been able to see the hairdresser. I've finally got an appointment for next Saturday. I like wearing my hair down to my shoulders... It's easy and comfortable. I think for me, it looks more professional. This is the most natural that my hair has been for ages. Since I haven't had the benefit of the hairdresser, it's like, "What do I do with it?" My middle daughter in particular, has helped as she can do all sorts of stuff with hair, but I haven't had any chemicals in my hair for ages.

My eldest daughter and my youngest daughter have different textured hair, so they can do many, many things. On the other hand, I find washing it is a chore, all the maintenance and the time it takes is a pain. My children laugh at me. But everybody's got their particular skill sets and I prefer going to the hairdresser to get my hair done.

Do you think the brands that sell products for Black hair could do more?

I think now, as compared to when I was growing up, there are a lot more brands. There's a lot more education too. I think Black people in particular, and especially young people, have accepted their natural hair, they're not trying to fit into some sort of stereotype, and as a result of that, they are now dictating what the market needs to prepare for them. Since they have done that, the market is now trying to catch up and it's a huge market. And because of that, there are a lot more products for different types of hair: curly, wavy and natural, and all of the stuff that I did not have access to. So I think it's amazing, that my children have all these options, as opposed to just saying, you're a Black person, and so this is what I'm going to give to you. I think that's a beautiful thing.

What do you think of products such as skin-lightening creams?

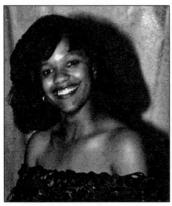

I thought it was objectionable back then, and I think it's even more objectionable now. I think we are a beautiful race of people, and we come in all different shades, color, creed, all of that. I think once you accept yourself for who you are, then you get confidence within yourself. Of course today you get bombarded by social media and all of that stuff telling you that you need to buy into all of these stereotypes, but I think if you have a strong foundation and someone is telling you that you have value and you are loved, then you can get past that.

You need to tell your kids that you are proud of them, and it's not so much about their accomplishments, but it's about the true essence of who they are.

Can you easily find products for your skin tone?

I don't really wear make-up, I never have. I think when I was growing up, I wanted to but my grandmother said, "If God wanted to give you eyes like that and pink cheeks, you would have been born like it," and then I had no interest. Unfortunately, it did not work with my children, but it worked with me...

What do you think the difference is between the way Black men and Black women are treated in society when it comes to standards of beauty?

The difference also comes from us because of the way we look at ourselves. The way we speak about ourselves, and also the perception we have of ourselves and that causes me pain sometimes. I speak about it to my kids, because they're the only people I have influence on. I want them to take a harder look and realize there is more to them than what other people see of them.

So what more needs to be done to empower Black women?

Black women need to realize that we are the most educated people on the face of the planet in every sphere of life. We need to own it and recognize the value that we have. We control so much, but then we give it away with our words.

We raise nations, but we also need to raise ourselves and hold ourselves with the highest esteem. We must look at and talk about ourselves with self-esteem. Additionally, we must hold those who are there to support and uplift us accountable. When they do anything but build us up and empower us, we need to see it as their fault and not our own.

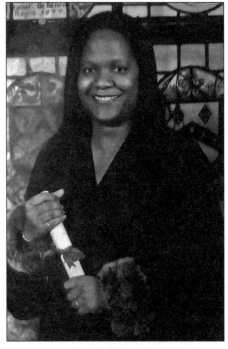

What advice would you give to your younger self today?

I would say: (A) Don't be so hard on yourself. (B) Learn to smile more. (C) It's going to all come out in the wash. I was way too serious. I would definitely tell myself to have a little bit more fun.

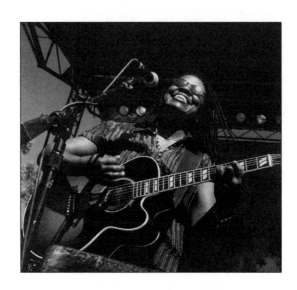

RUTHIE FOSTER

Ruthie Foster was born in 1964 and grew up in Gause, Texas. She was in the church choir singing solo by the age of 14, and subsequently went to college to study music and sound engineering. She then joined the Navy, where she performed with the Navy Band. After leaving the Navy, Foster moved to New York, where she began playing in folk clubs, eventually signing a deal with Atlantic Records. In 1993 she returned home to care for her sick mother for a few years, before resuming her music career and releasing her first album, *Full Circle,* in 1997. In 2010, her album *The Truth According to Ruthie Foster* received a Grammy nomination for Best Contemporary Blues Album. In 2012, *Live at Antone's* won the Blues Music Awards' DVD of the Year Award. Other notable awards include:

Contemporary Blues Female Artist of the Year 2010 (Blues Music Awards), Blues Artist of the Year (Female) 2010 (Living Blues Critics' Poll), Koko Taylor Award for Traditional Blues Female Artist of the Year 2011, 2012, 2013, 2015, 2016, 2018, 2019, and induction into the Texas Music Hall of Fame 2019 (Austin Music Awards).

What was your go-to hairstyle as a child, and who used to do your hair?

My hairstyle as a child was usually plaits with rubber bands and ribbons.

Who was your hair inspiration growing up? Did you struggle to find Black hair inspiration?

My hair inspiration came from magazines and TV in the 70s. Pictures of actors and poets like Cicely Tyson and Maya Angelou had a huge influence on me. Learning to braid was a necessary skill as a young Black girl.

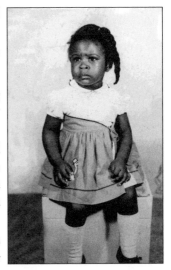

I was also envious of my older girl cousins who wore Afros to school everyday. Though my mother flat out refused to allow me to wear my hair in an Afro. She was a licensed beautician and insisted that my hair always stayed "put together" as she'd say. So she would wash and hot comb my hair regularly. The struggle was real!

Who are the Black female role models in society, and how do they differ from the role models you had growing up?

Well we have many! For me there's Oprah, Michelle Obama, Viola Davis, Venus and Serena Williams, Jada Pinkett Smith, Gayle King, Shonda Rhimes, Regina King, Beyoncé to Vice President Kamala Harris, all stand out as the epitome of Black women of power and so much more.

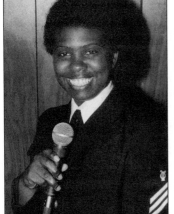

The only difference is that Black women are showing up as role models to all young girls, not just young girls of color. I think that's beautiful!

When you were young, what beauty standards did you associate with being beautiful, and how do they differ today?

Beauty standards for me were basically about not embarrassing my mother! Seriously though, growing up in rural central Texas as a young, traveling musician representing my church and family in the 1970s, the beauty standards were about looking as put together as you could possibly be; hair in place, dresses with pantyhose, modest jewelry etc. It was almost like a cruel joke that I was such a shy kid but was given this gift that required me to be an extrovert. So when I was told I looked 'pretty' it was usually only then that I felt that way. That's changed. I remind myself that I'm beautiful inside and out on a regular basis!

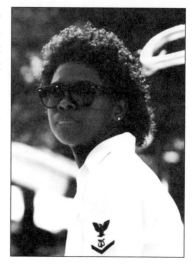

Can you remember when you were first made to feel like your hair was different? Tell us about that experience, what it felt like and how you navigated that?

I grew up aware that my hair was different. Starting with how much hair I had on my head! Having to sit in a kitchen on a hot Texas summer day while my mother washed my hair (twice!), conditioned, hot combed, styled with pink rollers and pins and wrapped my hair every Saturday afternoon.

What age were you when you started to make your own hair decisions, what were those decisions, and why did you choose the style you did?

I was about 13 years old when I started doing my own hair. I usually chose two braids with a split down the middle. I later got into braiding my hair regularly, thanks to my very skilled cousins on long bus rides after school.

What part does your hair play in your life today? What in your 'hair story' helped shaped that?

After many early years of processing my hair I choose to wear it in locs now for the past 20 years or so. I can still put it up in a ponytail or anything else. It's very comfortable and I love that it's natural and healthier.

What more do you think needs to be done to empower Black women, particularly regarding hair and beauty?

I think it's important for those of us who have lived the Black woman experience to share our stories and our trials with hair and beauty more often. It will only help and empower some young Black girl out there who is struggling right now.

What advice would you give to your younger self today? Or, what do you wish your younger self had known, that you know today?

I would tell little Ruthie that her experience is all part of a long, necessary and beautiful journey. So take notes so that you can help your own and so many other beautiful, Black daughters out there one day!

Anything else you want to say?

Love, peace and hair grease everybody!!

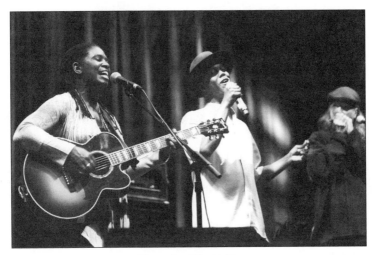

Photo: Jennifer Noble

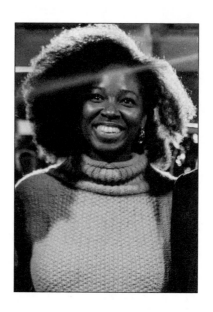

JAMELIA

Jamelia grew up in the Handsworth area of Birmingham. She signed her first major record deal straight out of school at 15. In 1999 she released her debut single, 'So High', followed by 'I Do' but her third single, 'Money', reached number five in the UK charts, winning her the Best Video gong at the 2000 MOBO Awards. In 2004, she had three more top-five hits, all from her album *Thank You*. Jamelia later returned to the Top Ten with the single 'Stop', her track for the second *Bridget Jones* film. Her continued chart success led to her being invited to support acts from the US, including Destiny's Child, Justin Timberlake and Usher, on their massive world tours. She has won four MOBO awards, including Best UK act and Best British Female. She has also performed at the MOBOS and co-hosted them in 2007. She has won a Q Award and has been nominated for 9 Brit Awards.

In 2008 Jamelia made her first documentary for BBC3, *Jamelia: Whose Hair Is It Anyway*, which looked at the hair extension industry, followed in 2011 with the BBC3 documentary, *Shame About Single Mums*. She was a TV presenter on *Loose Women* from 2103-16 and appeared on the BBC's *Strictly Come Dancing* in 2015.

Jamelia is also very active in her charity, working with ActionAid, the Princes Trust and the World Food Programme. Away from the spotlight, Jamelia still lives in Birmingham with her two daughters, Teja and Tiani.

What was your go-to hairstyle as a child, and who used to do your hair?

I'd say before the age of 10, I'd always have my hair in cornrows, and if it were a special occasion, I'd have a twist out, or I would have bunches in a twist. My hair kind of looked like how it is now, kinky. My mum's always been incredibly creative, so I'd always have the loveliest styles. She'd cut my brother's hair as well – she was like the barber for the area; all the boys in the neighbourhood would come and get their hair cut by her. I was known for my little hairstyles when I was younger. I'm Jamaican, so hair is a huge part of our identity. Until the age of seven, I had dreadlocks – my locks were down to my bum, and I wish I'd kept them now! I think a huge part of my identity was in my dreads. I was really proud of my Blackness and my African heritage – my connection to Africa. As a Jamaican, I didn't know any Africans growing up. I didn't know anyone who had been to Africa, so my connection was all through the history I was taught. My hair was connected to the warriors in Ethiopia, and it was a really important thing for me. I know that [if I'd kept the dreads], my life wouldn't have gone in the same direction it has gone, but I feel like I would have made some bold moves in my life. I remember myself at the time with dreads being really confident and free. You'd be walking down the street, and you'd see another Rastafarian and be like, "Irie." It was a language, but you had a real sense of community, and my hair was the outward indicator of it. I feel like a lot of things that happened after, are directly connected to coming away from Rastafarianism and the community that had been created.

Who was your hair inspiration growing up?

In my teen years, my biggest hair idol was my mum, but the problem with that was that my mum had a sort of Indian textured Afro hair, and people were always asking, "How come your hair is not like your mum's?" I would always try and emulate her curl pattern even after she'd relaxed my hair when I was about 10 – my mum's hair wasn't relaxed – so when I got to my teen years, that's when I started seeing other Black teens with relaxed hair. And that was from the TV: Moesha, *Sister, Sister,* Mary J. Blige, Aaliyah, TLC, SWV (Sisters With Voices), Jade – and that's when I started getting hair inspiration from like celebrities, and I got extensions like Jade. I had the SWV's particular style where they would swoop the front of their hair and then have braids on the top, like Cardi B did in a recent video – if you're an 80s child, then you know! All of my hairstyles were from music stars. So, one week it would be loads of bobbles like Da Brat – I even discovered a way to curl and pin my hair, so I looked like I had a small hairstyle without cutting it. But I feel like I got a huge portion of my inspiration when I was going to school. I'd be up at 5.00 am – I had to leave my house at 7.00 am, but I'd be up at 5.00 am because my hair had to be on point. I used to do this thing called a French roll, having ringlets going down the front. Mum always knew – buy me a curling tong, and I'd be in heaven! I remember wanting this tiny, tiny curling tong that could do little ringlets at the front. I was obsessed with my hair at school, and it wasn't like I wanted to do hair, I just liked my hair looking nice. I was known for my hair at a school. I was popping every day!

Did you struggle to find Black British hair inspiration?

Definitely, I feel like I didn't watch British TV at all until I started appearing on TV. I never watched *EastEnders* or other soaps. I didn't find the comedies funny. When I was 18, that was when I started watching *The Richard Blackwood Show*. We had the Ian Wright show, *The Real Mcoy* and Trevor Nelson's shows – we started to get shows, the older I got, and they were a part of my formative years. But even so, they were very male-dominated. I think Beverley Knight was the only Black woman who I thought was amazing, and I used to think I want to look like her, and I share and identify with her because of her complexion. She had short hair, and I'm sure I cut my hair around the time Bev was around. I feel like the girl groups we had at the time were knock-off versions of American artists, so my focus at the time was on Americans – it's a bit sad to think about. I've just started posting throwbacks on my Instagram. To hear people saying things like that [I'm an inspiration], it's just like, "Oh my God". For me, it was always the Americans, and to think I could become a person to have that kind of influence is amazing. And I love the fact that the space in which my daughters exist is very different now. I think we've got many examples – here and across the pond – of our beauty, and I love it.

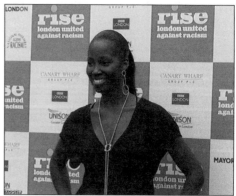

Jamelia at the Rise Festival, 2007

Who are the Black female role models in society, and how do they differ from the role models you had growing up?

I think the female artists and celebrities back then were told who to be and how to present themselves. It was implied that if you didn't comply, it wasn't going to work out. And I feel like a lot of record labels specifically went for Black people from inner cities, so we felt indebted to them and were more malleable because we didn't have money and money was being offered. I think about people like Janelle Monáe, Yara Shahidi, Tracee Ellis Ross, Alison Hammond, Judi Love. We can exist more unapologetically, and I think the more we have people [like them] pushing those boundaries, I feel like we're getting more variety. We're seeing ourselves in different ways, spaces and places, and that's exactly as it should be. Black women should be normalized. I still don't think we're as free as we could be when it comes to hair, but when it comes to visibility, I think it's the support of Black women that allows other Black women to be unapologetic despite the mainstream gaze, ideas and agendas. And then you see people like Viola Davis in *How to Get Away With Murder* – when I saw her take off her wig, I was like, "Oh my God", and when I saw her tie up her head, I was like, "Oh my God". I just thought it was revolutionary, and I was an adult seeing this, but what I love is that my daughters will watch this and just think this is normal. This is just TV. We support these things by our reactions, by being loud and being appreciative of these kind of visuals.

When you were young, what beauty standards did you associate with being beautiful, and how do they differ today?

After my Rasta foundation, I went to a pan-African Saturday school. These were really important events and experiences to have in my life, and I think they helped shape me. There were conversations that we were having then that we're having today about colourism and the optics when it comes to Africa about our identity and beauty. These things we were discussing at seven years old, this was my environment, this was my conversation, so I was very fortunate as a dark-skinned Black girl growing up to see myself as beautiful. Not only that, but when it comes from Rastafarianism, it's all based on love and loving everyone, and I was taught to appreciate the beauty in everyone and everything around me. Being told at 16 that I was too dark and I wouldn't be able to make it – I couldn't fathom why that would be a factor in whether or not I could be successful. I think that would have broken some people, but I was too confident about myself. I knew too much about myself – so whilst I definitely grew up being aware of Eurocentric ideals of beauty, I'd already been injected with a level of self-confidence that a lot of Black British children hadn't been and still aren't being injected with to this day. And that's sad.

Beauty standards to me had nothing to do with what you looked like because the beauty standards that I had been raised in were just: what type of a person are you? Are you good, bad, kind – those were the ways you judged a person's beauty, not whether or not they had light skin or curly hair. When I would see it in someone else or hear those conversations, I couldn't keep it to myself; I had to question it. For instance, I was really recognising how differently they would treat and approach my lighter-skinned daughter to my older, darker-skinned daughter. I remember feeling compelled to inject that sense of positivity and self-love into both of them. It felt like I was fighting against something else, and it's a strange experience when I didn't grow like that in an environment where that was a thing. Also, I didn't watch TV, so I wasn't receiving messages that my Blackness was anything other than beautiful, and I didn't know if that was intentional by my mum. I feel like I have been very intentional around my girls and the environment that I have allowed them to exist in.

At what age were you made to feel like your hair was different? Tell us about that experience, what it felt like and how you navigated that?

My first negative experience to do with my hair was when I was 35 – shocking, I know. I had relaxed hair from the age of 10, and before that, I had come from a really positive environment. After I big-chopped at 35, it was the first time I didn't tell anyone, and I didn't like it, so immediately I put my hair in braids for at least six months, and then after that, I went on *Loose Women*, and it was like I was debuting my new hair. I had two reactions: white women asking me, "What on earth have you done to your hair?" I had little twists at the front, and one of them asked, "Have you got snakes in your hair?" I was like, you lot are big women! I was shocked. It's a live show, so I had to go on because I had committed to it. But the reaction from Black women, oh my gosh, was so beautiful, and it totally counteracted the reactions I received from my colleagues or the people I was working with

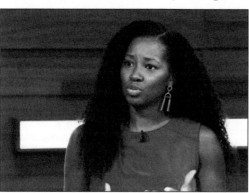

at the time, and I just felt so warm and thankful. So, the first time I got a reaction was when I decided to publicly wear my natural hair, but the Black women's reaction solidified that this was what I wanted to do.

Jamelia on *Loose Women* 2015

Do you have any experiences where your hair had a major effect on something in your life?

Yeah – returning to natural is when I first had any form of negative hair experiences. Around the same time in 2015, I went on to *Strictly Come Dancing,* and every week they said, "We need your hair to be straight, it cannot look like that – it's not elegant, it looks messy." This was every week for ten weeks. I would get this by email, I would get it over the phone, I would get it in person, and every week I would be in tears telling them: "Do you understand what you're saying to me? And not only to me, but you're also saying this to every Black girl who has hair like me.

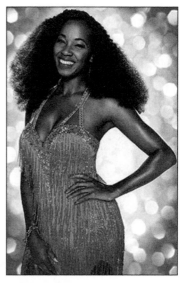

Why can't they watch *Strictly* and see somebody who looks like me, somebody with their hair?" I remember feeling like it was such a fight, just to exist in that environment. Black women understand just how important we are to the amplification and the normalisation of ourselves, our hair, our bodies. The more that we speak about it and celebrate it and promote it, the more normal it will become. And as someone who has been on the other side of the camera, it's important to speak on it. I was like, "Do you understand that this is a permanent chemical process that you're asking me to do to my hair?" By this time, I was balling. And every week, I went on with my hair out. They didn't have a make-up artist that could do Black skin, and they didn't have a hairstylist that could do Black hair, so I had to do my own hair and make-up every week. This is a show that goes out to millions of people every week, and then every morning, I'd go and sit in the make-up chair for them to take photos pretending that they had done my hair and make-up. And that year, they got a Bafta for Hair and Make-up, so I was like, "Oh, I won a Bafta," because I was on that team. I've built resilience; I feel like I've changed as a person, and I feel like all of these changes have been for the better, so I wouldn't have it any other way. Even my persona in the public eye – I'm so nonchalant. I'm not interested in the limelight or being famous. If I do something, it's because I want to do it, and if you mention my hair, just drop me out.

What part does your hair play in your life today?

My hair is a celebration of who I am and I love to see other women expressing themselves as well. I especially love seeing teens embracing and playing and being creative with their natural hair. And I've always made a point of telling little Black girls that their hair is beautiful and pointing out similarities, like when little Black girls come up to me and say, "Your hair is beautiful," I'll say: "Well, it's just like your hair, we've got the same hair!" And as much as I wouldn't wear a weave, I love to see people with it. Like, if you have blue hair, I'm like, "Yeah, man, you express yourself." Our hair is where we express our freedom, and because we are so varied because we are out and loud, and we're no longer hiding away and making it look 'presentable'. To me, that is just beautiful. There was a period when you had to look a certain way, and you had to tone it down, and I feel like the unapologeticness is contagious. I love it. The same way we have to speak out loud, we have to exist out loud, you know, put on your weave, put on your wig, put on your Afro – it's so beautiful for us to feel free to express ourselves authentically.

What do you think about how brands situate themselves in the narrative of Black hair? What more do you think could be done?

I feel like they use us for decoration. If they were serious about change, diversity, and progression, they would ensure they had us on their teams. That being said, I feel like it's a step in the right direction because we weren't even being included in the conversation before. Still, I don't feel like all racism is over because they've got a Black woman in the Pantene advert – no, make sure the products work, make sure you're not including chemicals that affect Black women, make sure our products work for us. There's so much more to be done. I feel that brands should be employing Black women to be consultants, and they're not – they're just employing Black women to be models, and they think that's enough. There are so many Black women who have different haircare ranges – I'm the type of person who always used to make my own hair care, and now I'm in contact with so many amazing Black women who make incredible products that are for us. They're natural, and they haven't got all of the sulphates; they're not mass-produced. I'd much rather spend my money there.

What more do you think needs to be done to empower Black women in terms of the beauty standards set for them?

I think it's about us normalising ourselves. It's about celebrating each other, the support of each other, being honest about our experiences and helping each other out. I feel like it's happening – Black women are the backbones of society, and I feel like the power lies with us, and as long as we recognize the power and the goddess in each and every one of us, then to me, we don't need anybody else. We are it.

What do you think of the differences between the way Black men and Black women are treated in society when it comes to standards of beauty?

There's definitely a divide. Black men are hugely fetishized, and Black women are also fetishized, but not in the way of wanting us; it's in the way of wanting to emulate or steal our attributes. So, it's OK to use Black women. Black men are being used as well, but they're adored in a way that Black women aren't – we aren't given credit for the impact that we have on society. I feel like we don't get our flowers, and that's why I say we need to make sure we give ourselves the flowers because, again, we can't be waiting on mainstream society to build up our self-esteem and self-worth. People like the Kardashians have really popularized that fetishisation, and they use our Black men, throw them away, take them back, and then degrade them. Their whole aesthetic is a Black female aesthetic, and I feel like that has really permeated the culture and begun to become a normal and accepted thing. Still, again it's for us, as Black women, to understand that whatever they're choosing to monopolize or appropriate does not take away from us.

What advice would you give to your younger self today? Or what do you wish your younger self had known, that you know today?

I wish I'd known how much beauty, power, influence, heritage and history was within my hair. I wish I'd known earlier to celebrate myself in my entirety because I think whilst I was extremely confident when I was a young girl and a teen, my hair was something I wasn't that proud of. Every six weeks, I was trying to get rid of the regrowth, and I wish I knew that it was going to be something that I celebrated and absolutely adored in years to come. It's given me so much in confidence and self-esteem because it's given me the ability to speak and exist out loud. So my advice to my younger self would be: don't dismiss any part of you.

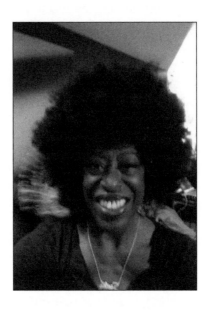

JUDITH JACOB

Judith has been a professional actress for over 40 years. She is the daughter of Grenadian parents, from Sauteurs and Gouyave.

Her first job was at the age of 13 for the BBC Play for Today *Jumping Bean Bag*. Since then, she has been consistently seen on television, from drama series, as nurse Beverley Slater in *Angels* (BBC), to comedy, as Sensimilla in *No Problem* (devized by the actors and written by Mustafa Matura/Farruk Dhondy who were all part of Black Theatre Co-op) for Channel 4, in *Eastenders,* as Carmel Roberts (BBC), in *The Real McCoy,* a sketch show playing various characters (BBC), as well as many other television programmes.

Judith had her own live chat show, *Judith Jacob Yabba Yabbas with Friends* which was very successful and featured various artists such as Janet Kay, Rudolph Walker, Kwame Kwei-Armah, Garth Crooks, Felix Dexter, Omar and many, many more.

Judith is one of the co-founders of The Bibi Crew, who wrote, produced and marketed their productions of *On A Level, But Stop! We Have Work To Do, Shutdown* and *Get Raunchy*. She is currently on Concious Radio 102fm every Thursday 1–4pm playing music and chatting to various guests.

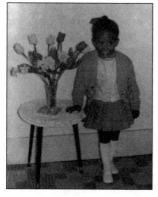

What was your go-to hairstyle as a child, and who used to do your hair?

My mum used to do my hair. I remember at around three years old wearing three plaits – one in the front and two in the back. Then it was two cornrows. At some point, my mother decided to straighten my hair with chemicals, i.e. hair straightener, before I went on a school holiday, which was a disaster because I didn't know how to care for it so my hair fell off at the back. My mum was convinced that someone had taken a pair of scissors to my head. Then it was back to the hotcomb. That was a constant fear that my ears would get burnt.

Who was your hair inspiration growing up? Did you struggle to find Black hair inspiration?

I never thought about who inspired my hairstyles as my mum made those decisions, however, I know I wanted flowing hair that fell on my face so that when I shook my head it would move from side to side. That probably meant any white female with long hair was what I wanted, or my mum's kind of hair. When I was 17, I was working on a TV show, *Angels,* and I wore my hair natural and it wasn't a conscious thought to find Black hair inspiration as cornrows and 'fros were prominent at that time, so that's what I did prior to me locksing my hair, which I had wanted to do in my late teens, but I was made to think that I would not get any acting work if I did.

Who are the Black female role models in society, and how do they differ from the role models you had growing up?

There is no one person, except maybe my mum. I get excited when I see intricate hair plaiting and cornrows, like the Ethiopian hairstyles. I absolutely love 'fros whether they are big or tiny. I should say my mother had long soft hair because her dad, my grandfather, who I never met, was an indigenous Grenadian which means his hair was the same texture as most Indian Asians.

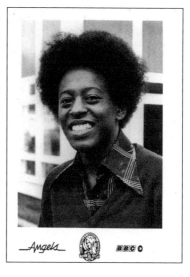

When you were young, what beauty standards did you associate with being beautiful, and how do they differ today?

The standard of beauty when I was young was anything that wasn't African. Straight nose, long flowing hair and not dark skin. Now, I am totally the other way from the time when I became educated about my rich, inventive, creative history. I so appreciate the texture of our African hair, the uniqueness, the growing to the sun. I love all of the shades of our Blackness from the caramel to the blue black.

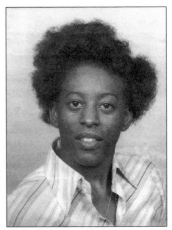

Can you remember when you were first made to feel like your hair was different?

I knew that it was different from my life at home as the hotcomb was part of my childhood. I didn't think my hair was bad just that it needed to be straight to make it 'manageable'. My younger sister's hair was more similar to my mum's so she got compliments from family members. I went to a primary school that had a lot of African Caribbean children so we bonded and I got strength from that – but it's only in retrospect I can say that.

What age were you when you started to make your own hair decisions, what were those decisions, and why did you choose the style you did?

I would say I made my own hair decisions at about 13 or 14. I remember doing Chiney Bumps (Bantu knots), then a Purdy hair style, taken from the *Avengers'* lead woman called Purdy, which meant I voluntarily used a hotcomb to straighten my hair and you couldn't sweat or all the straightness would go. I also rocked a 'fro which took time to manage and then you had to pat it down so no strand was sticking out. I was very much influenced by what was the fashion of the day. The 70s was very Black Power so I was in that style.

Do you have any experiences where your hair had a major effect on something in your life?

Not really. The biggest experience was me deciding to lock my hair as I had to hold my breath to see if I would work as an actress again but as there was so much ignorance about locks it didn't stop my career which I thought it might.

At that time, hair and make-up artists assumed that my locks were hair extensions. I remember being asked how long it took me to do my hair in the morning and I said I get up at 4 am to do my hair. That was a total lie but I just felt that I know all about your hairstyles and perms so you should know about mine. Bob Marley was extremely popular then so I was being asked what I felt was a stupid question therefore it did not deserve a decent answer.

What part does your hair play in your life today? What in your "hairstory" helped shaped that?

I love my hair. I play with it doing all kinda things with my locks. I have also got a beautiful Afro wig. If I didn't have locks I would twist it and sport all kinds of African styles as the beauty of our hair is endless. I have had a journey with my daughter's hair too which was straightened, then weaved and only three years ago did she finally embrace her natural hair. She wears extensions now but before that she was sporting a very short 'fro; so beautiful.

What do you think about how brands situate themselves in the narrative of Black hair? What more do you think could be done?

I am not too aware of brands that are not African-run as I have only used natural oils like coconut, almond. However I am totally aware that African women spend a good deal of money on their hair and anybody with any business sense would want the African/Black pound. What is being done now is that more African Caribbean people have set up businesses producing hair products that are not harmful to our hair.

Do you think there is a difference in the way Black men and Black women are treated in society when it comes to standards of beauty?

There is a big difference with how African Caribbean British men and women are treated. Firstly, a dark skin man is seen for his beauty which is not always the case for women. There is an expression: "a woman's hair is her beauty", which usually refers to straight, flowing hair, while men do not have that said

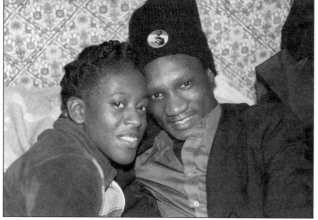

about them.

Black women are often compared to European beauty standards, unfairly.

What more do you think needs to be done to empower Black women, particulary regarding hair and beauty?

Children at primary school need to see images that represent themselves in all their glory. 'Fros, cornrows, extensions, wavy hairstyles and all the shades that we come in. I must say, there are a lot more books for children being published today that do offer that, and these books just have to make their way into the schools. We also need more images of African/Black women who are successful in their chosen fields, to see their beauty as not just skin deep, but that you can choose any profession your heart desires and European beauty ideals do not determine your success.

What advice would you give to your younger self today? Or, what do you wish your younger self had known, that you know today?

My younger self had a lot of confidence because my parents made me feel like I was all that! However I was very spotty in my early teens. I would let my younger self know nothing stays the same and what seems really painful now will become a distant memory and your pain will help you to grow. You will become desirable to many and not have to settle for less. Do not let the things that scare you stop you from doing it. Listen to yourself, use that intuition.

Anything else you want to say?

I believe I was bought up at a very political time in history. A 60s baby and even if I was too young to appreciate the Black Power Movement, The West Indian Cricket team, and the power of Muhammad Ali, they all affected my upbringing because they affected my parents.

My African learning didn't really start till I was 19 from an amazing man called Archie Poole. I dressed like a boy in my early years as I thought I wanted to be a boy. I think I must have realized that boys had more power and I didn't feel like boys would look at me – mainly because of my acne and my short hair which certainly was not deemed beautiful. I am the only child out of my siblings who took the same texture hair as my dad and somehow I knew that made a difference. However it's a difference that I love!

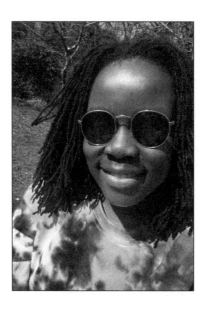

BAKITA KASADHA

Bakita Kasadha is a health writer, health researcher and poet. She works at the University of Oxford and has written for a wide range of publications, including *Glamour UK, Metro,* gal-dem, *Black Ballad* and the *British Journal of Healthcare Management.* She grew up in Eltham (Greenwich borough), and as a teenager often travelled to Lewisham and Southwark for hair products and to get her hair done.

What was your go-to hairstyle as a child, and who used to do your hair?

As a kid, the early part of primary school, my mum would section my 4C hair into four big plaits. It was manageable and functional. Some of the other kids at school called me "four planets" though. Now, they weren't bullying, it wasn't that, but it was teasing. It was frustrating and made me feel really visible in the worst way. After a while, I'm not sure how long, I told my mum to stop doing my hair like that. So then I tried to brush it down and keep it contained with hair clips, that really weren't designed with my hair in mind.

Growing up, I always felt like my hair was a hassle. Sometimes an emotional hassle and sometimes a painful one. Whenever it was box braided or cornrowed, all I would hear is "beauty means pain". I know I wasn't the only little Black girl to hear those words growing up!

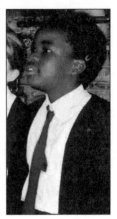

Who was your hair inspiration growing up? Did you struggle to find Black hair inspiration?

I can't remember many hair inspirations specifically, but they all had straight hair. I remember that my hair was blown-up and hot combed for my auntie's wedding, and it was the first time I truly loved my hair. I was around seven years old. From that moment until my teens I really wanted straight hair and tried my best to recreate that look with hot combs and relaxer.

Who are the Black female role models in society, and how do they differ from the role models you had growing up?

I think there are way more Black women in Britain on our screens now, than when I was growing up. That being said, I found so much joy in Angellica Bell on the TV screen. Still, her hair was straight, and I completely understand why.

When you were young, what beauty standards did you associate with being beautiful, and how do they differ today?

White women and slim. And that was a struggle, because I've had hips since puberty and I'll never be anything other than Black. I never saw myself as attractive, pretty or beautiful. Today? That's completely different and has been different for a number of years. I know generally there's been a movement, but I think the way I saw myself started to change in my late teens because I started to hang around more Black people and different races more generally. I was very intentional about going to Christ the King Sixth Form College, in South London for that reason. If only for two years, I didn't want my identity to be "the Black one".

At what age were you made to feel like your hair was different? Tell us about that experience, what it felt like and how you navigated that?

For as long as I remember until around Year 4, I was the only Black girl in my school and one of three Black kids. I knew I was different early on and envied the white girls with long straight hair. Sometimes I wonder if it was wanting to have the hair – well, I do think it was a lot to do with that – but I also think it was a lot about just wanting to fit in, if I'm honest.

When I was young, in my bedroom, I used to put the neck opening of T-shirts or jumpers around the crown of my head and pretend it was flowing hair. I used to swish the material around and pretend I had long 1C locks.

When I was still in primary school, I went to Uganda, where I'm originally from and had my hair braided with cornrows and white and red beads (matching my school summer dress). I loved it, especially because I could now swish my hair and beads. It's funny because now I have sisterlocks that pass my shoulders. I could 'swish' them, but I don't.

What age were you when you started to make your own hair decisions, what were those decisions, and why did you choose the style you did?

I think my hair was first relaxed when I was seven or eight years old. It's something that I'd asked for, and if I'm honest, nagged for! After that point, for upkeep my auntie would relax any new growth. I used to wet my hair in the bath to recreate that 'first relax' look. I'm sure it was awful for my hair – I was washing it way too much! It broke in my mid-teens.

Do you have any experiences where your hair had a major effect on something in your life?

Before I got locked, my loctician asked me if having sisterlocks would have a negative impact in my relationships, family life, work environment and religion. I am not sure what she would have said, had I replied "Yes", but it really got me thinking how wanting to simply embrace my natural hair could be seen negatively.

How do you wear your hair at work? Or for interviews? Has this changed over time?

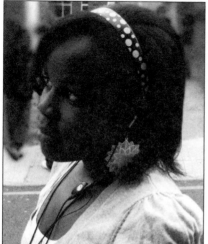

I have had sisterlocks since February, 2015. I usually have my hair down. I really need to be more adventurous with styling it (I have said that for at least three years)! But I love that it looks good without much effort. Before I used to blowout my hair and pull it back, anything to make sure it didn't stand out. I worried it would be distracting in interviews.

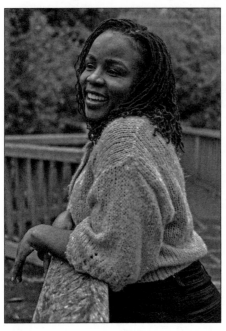

What part does your hair play in your life today? What in your "hair story" helped shape that?

I love my hair. I love that I have a natural, low-maintenance hairstyle. Towards the end of university, I started to 'experiment' with my hair. I wore my hair out: Afros, blow outs, braid outs. It was the first time in several years that I saw my hair as 'done' and believed that it being out was a hairstyle! Because I had more time at uni', I also box-braided my hair a lot, so for a few years I didn't hear that my hair was "tough" or difficult (by hairdressers). I learned how to comb my hair in a way that it didn't hurt too.

What do you think about how brands situate themselves in the narrative of Black hair? What more do you think could be done?

Honestly, I don't pay much attention to this. I seek out Black-owned brands and pretty much leave it at that.

What do you think of beauty products such as skin-lightening creams?

I'm glad I didn't even venture into that world. I am dark-skinned, but I think growing up in such a white area meant that I was bothered about my Blackness, rather than my darkness. I'm not sure if that makes sense, but dark/light skin didn't feature, it was more about being Black.

One time I went into a hair shop – you know those hair shops that double up as cosmetic shops. I asked for body oil and the owner took me to the aisle with a wide range of skin-lightening creams. Most of them had South Asian women on the covers, with a clearly photoshopped version of them with different skin tones. I never went back to that shop. It's annoying, because this shop stocked aisles and aisles worth of body products and creams, for all different purposes. The fact that that shop owner looked at me and immediately thought I wanted lightening cream was a shit feeling.

Can you easily find beauty products which suit your skin tone?

Yes. Thanks to the internet!!!

What do you think of the differences between the way Black men and Black women are treated in society when it comes to standards of beauty?

Black men are fetishized and features commonly attributed with Black women, are fetishized on non-Black women. I think we're at opposite ends of a perverse spectrum in many ways and it's not good for either of us.

What more do you think needs to be done to empower Black women, particulary regarding hair and beauty?

It needs to start when we're girls. We need to affirm our baby girls' hair. I wrote a poem called *I am not woke*, and a line in it says: 'our hair defies gravity and yes, there's magic in that. Our hair grows towards the life force – yes, there's power in that. In its natural state, our hair gives us a standing ovation – there's adoration in that'.

We need to drum into them that the way their hair grows isn't a political statement. It's beautiful. There's nothing wrong with our hair and everything wrong with anti-Black racism.

What advice would you give to your younger self today? Or, what do you wish your younger self had known, that you know today?

Beauty doesn't mean pain. Beauty means comfort, it means celebration, it means calm. You'll grow to love your skin. You will learn to adore your hair. You will be so proud to be Black that it'll shock you, but it's going to be such a beautiful surprise.

Anything else you'd like to add?

I don't know when I first came across sisterlocks, but when I did I knew that I would want that hairstyle. It took me about 18 months from wanting it, to getting it though. In that time, and years before, I was regularly getting my hair braided in a salon in Woolwich. Over the years, every professional doing my hair, has *always* commented on how "tough" my hair was. This includes hairdressers in south-east London all the way to hairdressers in Uganda! It broke combs, it was too thick. I remember one time, when I kinda embraced my natural hair – I say 'kinda' because it was natural and I was committed to that, but I always braided. But I remember a time when the person who braided my hair in Woolwich persuaded me to texturize my hair to "soften it". This was very much about her ease with my "tough hair". I told her that I wanted to keep my natural hair and she stressed that it would only soften it, it wouldn't change the structure. I agreed – bear in mind that she had been wearing me down for months. I used to go to her every two months. My hair texture completely changed, it was like it had been relaxed. I wish I had known more about hair products generally. I was devastated!

She also persuaded me to get a weave that day. I think she couldn't be bothered with the box braids anymore to be honest! Now I know it's not wise to have your hair texturized and weaved on the same day. I ended up with a bald patch on my scalp. We've really been through it, my hair and I. I took out the weave after two weeks, because my head was hurting so much and there it was – the bald patch. It had implications for when I finally got my sisterlocks, because my loctician had to cut off all the texturized bits. I was probably left with half to a third of my original length.

My loctician is the only professional who has ever celebrated my hair. I have had locks for just over six years and I will also remember when she called my hair "perfect" for sisterlocks. She called it "full" and "strong" and really helped me to have more pride in my hair. Thank you, Michelle!

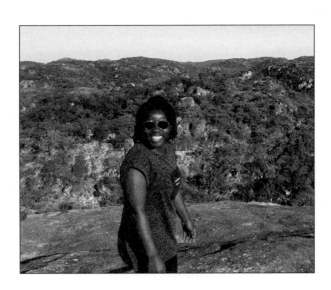

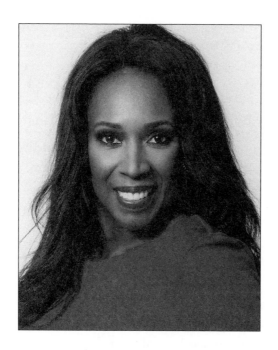

ANGIE LE MAR

Born in 1965 to Jamaican parents, Angie grew up in the London borough of Lewisham. After joining the Second Wave Women's drama group and attending stage school, she started working as an actress but dyslexia made it difficult for her to sight-read scripts. She thus decided to become Britain's first Black stand-up comedienne. In 1994, her debut comedy show *Funny Black Women on the Edge* scored a great success at the Edinburgh Fringe and was subsequently staged at the Theatre Royal, Stratford East whilst her self-penned series *The Brothers'* was produced on radio, TV and on stage. In addition to her work, she is the managing director of Straight to Audience Productions, where she writes and produces creative work.

What was your go-to hairstyle as a child, and who used to do your hair?

It's like we didn't even have a choice. It was: "Get here, your hair needs plaiting, your hair needs washing," and it's almost like my hair belonged to my mum really. So my go-to hair was always simple plaits. Just get in there, Mum and plait. I loved when my mum used to do Chiney Bumps (Bantu knots) when she washed my hair. Because the way my hair would open out afterwards, I used to think, that's the style, let me go now, but it was always, "No, we're just Chiney Bumpin' it, for now, when you're dry, we'll comb it out, and we'll plait it back again." I liked the actual Chiney Bumps (Bantu knots) because it's not like today where they've styled it; ours was just all over the place. So, I would put my hair in one, put in a little clip and go to school. Or I used to sleep with my hair in one and wake up thinking I'll just brush it like I didn't know I was Black, do you know what I mean? Those were the times when my mum would say, "Look how your hair knot up. Now we've got to undo it." And she just used to do it again. So, I couldn't even get away with that.

So, I look back on those times and think they were supposed to be cherished moments, but they weren't; let's not pretend. Although I used to like when the oil went into my scalp because that was very soothing, you know the Dixie Peach, and all of those oils going in felt like, "Oh right, that just kind of healed the bruises that she put through with the comb." It was very soothing the oil, definitely.

Who was your hair inspiration? And did you struggle to find inspiration?

Anybody at school who looked like they didn't struggle with their hair was my inspiration. If it looked like it could brush easy, without it being a trauma, that was it. Then growing up, when I started to see more hairstyles, if you had long hair, then we admired you. And if you weren't mixed raced and you were Black and had long hair, we looked at you like: "Wow! You've got long hair, and you're Black!"

When we saw hair on TV, it would be the American styles we wanted – that was another world over there, and it made us think, "Oh, there are alternatives we could have." Watching that in the 80s and 90s on TV and seeing Black

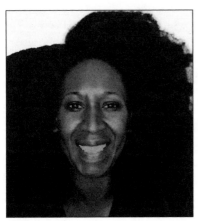

women doing the same hairstyles that we only saw on white women here was a real eye-opener that our hair could be as versatile.

We were watching programs, like *Charlie's Angels, The Cosby Show* or Debbie Allen from *Fame*, it was like watching a different world. We wanted our hair to move, so we'd put a cardigan or a towel on our head and flick it back and forth. When I used to make jokes and do stand-up about it, people would come up to me later and

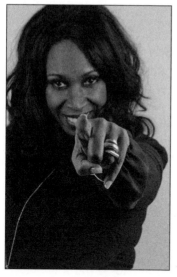

say, "Yeh, I did that." As if it was an unspoken thing we never talked about. I'm serious.

Who are the Black female role models in society today? How are they different to those you had growing up?

I grew up in the church, so for me, my role models were in the church. My mother was an evangelist, and there were great women leaders. There were powerful Black women who looked boss all the time. They were just suited and booted, and everything looked great. But as I got older and started watching the comedians, back in the day, the Whoopi Goldbergs, the Oprah Winfreys, those women were important. I learnt how to have my picture taken by copying Diahann Carroll. I used to flick through the magazines, *Ebony* and *Jet*, and all of those back in the day. Diahann was always poised really well and just looked absolutely beautiful. So, I always used to pose for pictures just like her and smile a little bit, just like she did. They influenced us and showed us that we could be, feel, look and say and do what we wanted.

Our catalogue of Black women now is so vast that it would be difficult for anybody to say that they can't see themselves in today's society. And though we might not be on television every day, there is a young Black girl somewhere who will go, "I want to do stand-up comedy", and she can find me, Gina Yashere, Judi Love – the list is endless. So when I look around I'm empowered by the variation of Black women, and I have a problem with people who think that we should be one way.

I think there's a quiet code that we have: we're trying to work each other out through our hair, because men dated us through our hair. If you had mixed-Indian hair, you could probably get a guy who has straight hair, or if you're light-skinned and you've got that type of hair. But if you're dark-skinned and your hair is thick, your children's hair will be short; I mean, that's what the 70s and the 80s were about.

When you were young, what beauty standards did you associate with being beautiful? So, what was your definition of beauty standards?

I started using anti-ageing cream at 19, because I went into a shop, and there was a Black woman there, and she said, "Angie, don't wait until your old to use anti-ageing cream and don't get into this notion that Black don't crack."

I'm 56 this year, so I'm all about, "How can I keep what I've got going?" Skin and teeth are my thing because that is the thing that ages you.

I wake up and I see myself, and I think, "You're just so awesome." I tell myself that, and I believe that, and I don't let people get to me. If I've been let down, I leave it in God's hands, as the bible says: "Vengeance is mine, says the Lord," and I leave it there. I get on with my day. So, when people go, "But weren't you upset?" Yes, I was upset, but I'm not going to let that define me. I've got things to do, and that's a distraction. I've got to look after myself, my three children and four grandchildren, one on the way. I actually won. Because to me, that's what success is. And the way I feel about myself inside is – I don't have a self-hate button, even when I don't feel well. Even when I'm overweight, and I feel like if I don't feel good in my body or whatever, I just go, "But I'm still here." Every day I wake up, and I go, "What else can you do? What else can you still do in this time?"

At what age were you made to feel like your hair was different? Tell us about that experience, what it felt like and how you navigated that?

I think early at school, I recognized that our hair is different, but it didn't make me feel less. When I was plaiting my daughter's hair when she was a child, I'd say, "I love this cornrow that I'm doing, you're going to love it," and she'd be sitting there like, "Just hurry up." And that's when I realized that this is what my mum went through. When I was coming into my teens, it was the boys that kind of defined us. Girls who were going out with guys were straightening their hair, so that's what we'd do too.

I had locs for eight years, but I had to cut them off because my hair was getting thin because of the dye, having it red all the time. So, when I cut it off, I put my hair in weave because it grows better. But people were telling me, "I don't like weave." I felt like saying, "Well then, don't wear it. Just leave me alone and don't judge me." I'm here to be funny; I'm not here for my hairstyle.

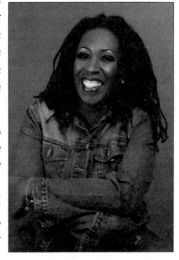

What age were you when you started to make your own hair decisions, what were those decisions, and why did you choose the style you did?

I used to have my hair in two cornrows when I was in my teens, and I wanted to press my hair, so I used to get an iron and literally iron it –

just stupidness. When I got to about 16, my mum let me perm my hair, but before that, we'd get 'Dark and Lovely', and my mates would come up in my bedroom, and they'd say, "OK, take it out now," and I'd say, "No don't take it out. I want it to be really straight." They'd say, "No, you've got to take it out now, it's starting to burn." Then you wash it out, and you've got this silky straight hair, and you think, "Wow, look at me!" And I remember putting in curlers and having it flicked up all the way around and just thinking: "I'm so gorgeous. Like I'm going to be inundated with men now because my hair is flicked up." But the thing was, it didn't stay, so by the time you got to a party, it would just flop, and you'd think, "This wasn't the plan."

Then I used the glue and watched my hair come off with it. You'd put a clamp in your hair, roll it on and clamp it. So, you had all these little metal clamps in your hair, which would turn your hair green. They didn't tell you that you couldn't wear the clamps for two or three weeks in a row. We kept them in for months, and then when you take them out, your hair is rusted green.

Have there been any experiences in your life relating to your hair that have had a major effect on you?

Not really. I think as you get older, you don't care as much. You just kind of get to a place where you enjoy who you are. There was a time when I wouldn't be out in the street without make-up or great hair. But I think as you get older, you worry less about fitting in. People actually have to fit in with you. When I was out there doing comedy back in the day, there were no Black women – I was the first. So, if you wanted a Black person and a woman, I was two for one. I was always ticking the boxes, so I was under this pressure to be really good or else the people behind me would struggle even harder. And after you've proven yourself in life, how long do you keep proving yourself for?

What do you think about the way brands situate themselves in the narrative of Black hair and what do you think needs to change?

I remember when my aunts used to send me Afrosheen in those little triangle bottles, and now you walk into a hair shop, and it's like, "What *don't* you have?" What I love is that it's Black women who are creating the products now. Verona White is my hair stylist/hair doctor, whose products, Afro Hair Growth Challenge, has seen my hair grow in ways I never expected, especially after I cut my locs.

I'm very careful now, and believe that if a brand isn't behind us, we shouldn't be buying it, simple as that. The Asian shops are so nice now because they realize that people are spending their Black pound there. They want our money, they want us to wear their clothes because they look good on us, they want our dance moves. White women want to copy our style, to wear hair extensions. Nobody says they're weird. So, we have a great brand as Black women, and we need to endorse each other and keep lifting each other up.

What do you think of the difference between the way that Black men and Black women are treated in society when it comes to standards of beauty?

I think we all know, for years, we have been fighting for balance and the right imagery. America has always been ahead of us, but that has a lot to do with numbers and history. It first comes down to breaking stereotypes of what a Black man or woman should be, and today we have made great progress; we are such a varied people. The pressure for Black men to be strong and exotic and not show emotions can have a damaging effect on them. Then we have the forever stereotype of Black women being strong and able to take the world on. No. We need to be seen as sensitive too. The sexual side to us rarely has any layers to how we feel.

It's also very lazy to see us as aggressive, while other women are seen as assertive and confident when they stand up for themselves; it is extremely wearing and problematic. We are forever trying to negotiate the room, and making others understand that yes, I was angry for that thing but no, the other thing was you, projecting your insecurities on me. We know we are beautiful [and through] the suntans, the lip fillers, the breasts, and the bums, society keeps showing us that – they are giveaways.

What more do you think needs to be done to empower Black women?

When I would have meetings in the past, they would never understand the stories I wanted to tell. If I had a comedy idea about successful Black women living a middle class lifestyle, they couldn't fathom that. They wanted trauma, they wanted our pain. If we are going to have trauma, we need balance; we are women whose experience is broad. We need happiness and laughter too. We have great writers like Michaela Coel, and those stories have to be told. But we have so many more stories in us, and making sure that we express them in theatre and film is a must!

In the 80s, I didn't think Black women got cancer because all the adverts were aimed at white middle class women. We had to campaign to say, can we have some Black women in those adverts because we are not checking our breasts because we can't see ourselves, and then we get diagnosed with cancer, and we die. Representation is important. If I see myself checking [in adverts], I'll check. So, I think we're moving nicely down that road right now. We must make sure that we are not being distracted by what people think we are fighting for. We are constantly rejected for how we want to portray ourselves by TV and the media. But social media is another powerful way, and we are addressing many of our issues with a true voice. The days of the weak narrative have gone because we control the pen. All our stories are important.

What advice would you give to your younger self today? Or, what do you wish your younger self had known, that you know today?

I would say: "You were right." I was kicked out of school because I'm severely dyslexic. I was the class clown, but look who I became? I became Britain's first Black stand-up, female comedian.

I would say to my younger self, "Everything that you're going through, you need it all. Enjoy it. Don't beat yourself up, don't go into any dark places where you start thinking: "Is it worth it?" Yes, it is. There will be good days, and there will be bad days, but more good than bad."

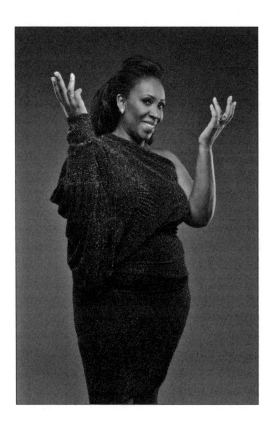

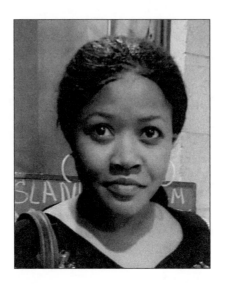

FRANCINE MUKWAYA

Francine Mukwaya is originally from the Democratic Republic of Congo (DRC) but now lives in Cambridge. She has been a human rights activist for 10 years, an event organizer, public speaker, member of the "support committee of Doctor Mukwege (2018 Nobel prize winner) in the Diaspora," and a political analyst (with a focus on the Great Lake region/Africa).

Born in Kikwit, a city in the western part of Congo, that is close to Kinshasa, the capitol city of DRC, Francine also works with the local community in Congo, especially internally displaced people, through *Kitunga ya mboka* (meaning Basket of the Country in Lingala language) an organisation in Congo. She started raising awareness of the on-going crisis in Congo several years ago and has appeared in the media, both in French and English, nationally as well as internationally. Francine has also written articles about the crisis in Congo and the conflict over minerals.

She has a BSC honours degree in Psychology and Counselling, a Masters degree in Public Health and a diploma in International Development. She says she is "allergic to injustice" and is passionate about women being empowered to change society. She also wants to see better health care provision for everyone as she believes that health is the key to the development of any society; when people are healthy, they are more able to reach their potential.

What was your go-to hairstyle as a child, and who used to do your hair?

My go-to hairstyle as a child was braided locks or adorned puffs. My mum used to do my hair most of the time but sometimes my mum's best friend who had a small salon. We used to go there once or twice a month.

Who was your hair inspiration growing up? Did you struggle to find Black hair inspiration?

My inspiration was M'bilia Bel, a very popular Congolese singer. She is an African legend. Growing up in Kikwit city in the western part of the Democratic Republic of Congo (DRC), a vibrant city not far from the capital where people love a mixture of traditional and modern music, M'bilia Bel was someone that most women or girls loved to see on TV, with her different hairstyles. Many women got inspiration from her and me and my mum would be listening or watching her on TV all the time at home. That made me want to copy her hairstyles. In Congo, we have many hairstyles which are nice, clean and acceptable, some are traditional hairstyles which have been modernized a bit. The struggle started when I moved to UK as I realized Black hair tends to have some sort of issue there in terms of keeping your hair natural.

Who are the Black female role models in society, and how do they differ from the role models you had growing up?

For me, personally, growing up in Congo, my role models were always my

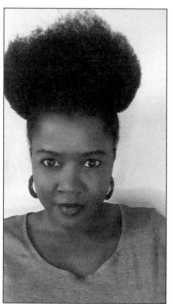

mother, my aunts, my grandmother and other women in Congo. These women carried on working even in difficult times. For instance, I used to see Congolese women, even in the middle of war, they'd wake up early morning, and go to the market to sell goods just to keep the family going. I would say my role models beyond my family have always been women in the civil rights movement or women fighting for peace and justice around the globe. Women such as Rosa Parks, Angela Davis and Kimpa-Vita (in Congo) and Queen Yaa Asantewaa (in Ghana).

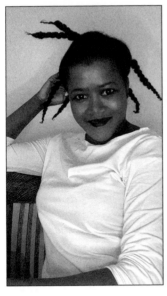

At what age were you made to feel like your hair was different? Tell us about that experience, what it felt like and how you navigated that?

I didn't have any problems until I was about 12 years old, when almost all my friends relaxed their hair. It was a bit of a shock and I was asking myself, "Why should I relax my hair?" So, one of my friends wanted to fit into the group, and I went with her to the local salon. While I was there, I could see the pain on her face, as she had the relaxer applied to her hair. But her mum was like, "Keep your head straight, let the hairdresser relax your hair." This got me questioning myself, seeing how my friend was in pain. It took me months to accept relaxing my hair but eventually I did. It was not an easy decision, because inside me I felt that it was wrong and when I grew up I was not going to do this to my hair.

What age were you when you started to make your own hair decisions, what were those decisions, and why did you choose the style you did?

When I moved to the UK, I was still relaxing my hair but it wasn't painful the majority of the time. I used a regular relaxer such as Dark and Lovely for a little while until, in 2010, I noticed my hair became very dry and thin. Then I decided to cut all my hair off and stayed with short hair for a while wearing wigs from time to time or braiding my hair. Inside me, I already knew that I wasn't going to relax my hair anymore. I feel like I made a very good decision; my hair is one part of my body and I need to care for it.

Do you have any experiences where your hair had a major effect on something in your life?

Yes I went for a job interview and I remembered one interviewer asking me, "Is that your usual hairstyle or do you straighten your hair as well?" He said, "It would look good if I straightened my hair." I told him, "I can't as it is just like someone asking me to straighten my eyes, my intestine or even my fingers." I said, "My hair is in its natural state as any other part of my body." They offered me a job but I refused it because I didn't feel comfortable working there. That was in 2012. Since then, I have become more conscious about Black hair.

How do you wear your hair at work? Or for interviews? Has this changed over time?

As someone who can't really sit two to three hours braiding my hair which I found difficult, I usually tie my hair back or on top of my head. I haven't really changed my hair style much. I have a big Afro that I do wear to work almost daily. I do braid my hair as well but not so often. Over time I learned to take care of my hair myself. I do my own hair mask, oil etc., and do my own Bantu knot when I am home.

What part does your hair play in your life today? What in your "hair story" helped shape that?

As a human rights activist and political analyst (with focus on Great Lake Region of Africa), I am often in front of the camera maybe doing interviews or attending conferences. Many younger activists, especially girls from that region have come to me and thanked me for inspiring them. In countries such as Congo for instance, buying Brazilian or Asian hair costs a lots of money. People have a choice to do whatever they want with their hair. However the pressure girls get to have those weaves is huge and it cost a lots of money. Seeing some Black women who are public speakers being able to wear their natural hair freely in front of the cameras has a huge impact. It's even fantastic when you hear them talking about it, or thanking you. That is "a story" that is shaping our community. For me, today, I believe that my hair plays an important role in this by making sure that people come to accept their hair as they have accepted other parts of their body.

What do you think of beauty products such as skin-lightening creams?

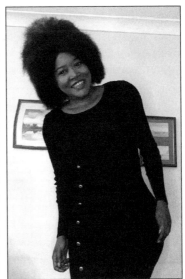

There is no health benefit to bleaching your skin. Lightening your skin can result in so many serious side effects and complications. Where I am from I've seen people around me such as my cousins, aunts etc. bleaching their skin to fit in. Knowing how skin bleaching reduces productivity of melanin in the skin, my dad was very strict on that and he used to tell us how he married my mum who has a beautiful dark skin. Skin bleaching is something that has a big health impact on people. It should be banned. I am glad some countries have banned the use of creams containing hydroquinine. But there is still a long way to go because people are still doing it and taking risks even though they know the impact. *The Guardian* published an article on how "Skin-lightening creams are dangerous – yet business is booming. Can the trade be stopped?" (April 2018). It is a very interesting article that people need to read.

Can you easily find beauty products which suit your skin tone?

Personally, it is a bit difficult as someone who has oily skin and where I live, there are not many shops that give me choices. I usually go down to London if I need to buy face cream. As someone who is considered to be a Key worker (in the health and social care industry), I was working the whole time during lockdown. Around May to July last year I had a break out on my skin that I had never experienced before. This was terrible and it was even worse wearing masks almost all the time at work. Then there was the issue of finding a face cream for my skin type. I used almost everything, I bought so many online but there was no solution until I went on YouTube and started looking at some videos. Rihanna's Fenty Beauty helped me out, especially Total cleanser and Hydra Vizor, and I also got Skin Clearing Serum Vitamin C+ by Eva Naturals. Regarding skin products, things need to improve because most of the face creams out there don't represent all skin types. They need to improve on this in terms of inclusion.

What do you think of the differences between the way Black men and Black women are treated in society when it comes to standards of beauty?

Society tends to hold the stereotype of Black men being aggressive, strong and to some extent, highly sexualized. I think it is by these standards that most Black men are judged or perceived. I feel like it is more about Black men's sporting ability and their sex appeal. Whereas, I feel like Black women are considered as strong women who can cope with anything. But if you voice your opinion then you are seen as an angry Black woman. Also the imposition on Black women to look a certain way, just to get a job or be treated as a professional or even to be accepted in society.

What more do you think needs to be done to empower Black women, particulary regarding hair and beauty?

Social media platforms have really contributed to normalising Black hair or Afro hairstyles. Although there is improvement, more needs to be done especially in mainstream media and the beauty industries. We need more Black women in the media, and journalists, wearing their natural hair because I believe representation is one of the solutions to what Black women face in terms of beauty standards. An example is when Zozibini Tunzi won the title of Miss Universe in 2019, her photos were shared all over Instagram and other social media, and this inspired a lot of young Black girls globally. I saw the shift and empowerment in so many social groups. This will help build more acceptance of your hair as part of your body and build self-confidence.

What advice would you give to your younger self today? Or, what do you wish your younger self had known, that you know today?

I'd tell her not to believe an answer is better than a question, to understand more about patience, and to remember that it is OK to be different and unique because your uniqueness is your power. I'd also tell her that it is OK to make mistakes because everyone fails big before they make it big. I would tell her to chase her passion and what she believes in relentlessly and not be afraid to ask lots of questions. In addition, I'd tell her that, no matter the judgement regarding how you look or perceive things, climbing Mount Kilimanjaro or Virunga may be hard but the view from the top of Kilimanjaro (Kenya) or Virunga (Congo) is divine.

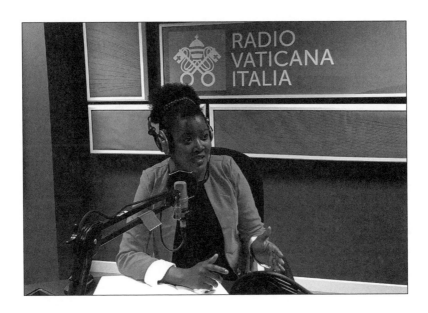

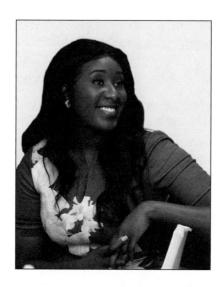

JESSICA OKORO

Jessica Okoro is an award-winning Business Consultant. Having started her philanthropic journey as a student, after overcoming struggles with her dyslexia to learn using traditional teaching methods in class, she developed her own learning resources and informal methods at home to achieve higher than expected exam results.

After her university degree, she went on to found BeScience STEM, a multi-award-winning charitable organisation which encouraged the whole community to engage in STEM, using innovative and creative techniques. Her charity has since had over 1000 volunteers and has engaged with 10,000+ people in the community within the first few years.

She has also worked as a consultant with various F-T100 companies such as Google, O2, HSBC. Her work has also been endorsed and supported by the likes of Presidents, Vice Presidents and Prime Ministers globally.

Her experience and knowledge have enabled her to guest talk and share her ideas about overcoming learning difficulties and the challenges for girls in STEM worldwide. As well as managing her charity, she works as a consultant for other charities and small organisations.

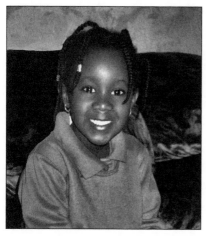

What was your go-to hairstyle as a child, and who used to do your hair?

Parting my hair into two and then tying the hair on the two sides, with pompoms. When I was a little older, I was more adventurous and would add a quiff at the front.

If not this look, I would have braids, which I hated the process of having done. Sitting in someone's home, with my neck resting between their thighs for four to six hours. Talking about life, family, troubles and celebrations. It was a love/hate process. What I did love was the intimacy, meeting people's family members and knowing you'd get a decent home-cooked meal mid-process.

The worst part of getting braids was taking them out and having neck cramps, keeping your head in the same position as you had to use the tail comb to take out each plait. It was a tedious task and very demotivating when I'd take out the braids and feel my hair hadn't grown a single inch. In some cases, it looked like it had even lost some inches.

Who was your hair inspiration growing up? Did you struggle to find Black hair inspiration?

I didn't have hair inspiration. All the women I saw on TV and in the media had extensions in and the Afro look wasn't exciting for me.

However, my mum used to take me to a phenomenal Afro Caribbean salon in Angel Edmonton, called Pamper Me. It was owned by one of my mum's close friends, late, Aunty Claudette. This was where I learnt about womanhood. It was a community of successful African Caribbean women from different walks of life: lawyers, mayors, business owners, wives, grandparents, who would, without fail, have their hair treatments every three weeks. Being surrounded by such women, gave me an early insight into Black female independence, striving to make your own money, looking after oneself and looking after your family. Although I would just go to get my hair braided for school, I felt this community hub was a second home, it was a sanctuary, a safe space for Black women.

I've yet to find another salon like this.

When you were young, what beauty standards did you associate with being beautiful, and how do they differ today?

When I was younger, I saw beauty only from a visual aspect, how a person looks and what they wear. But now, for me, beauty is confidence, someone embracing and knowing themselves well enough to do what their heart desires; not caring about society's standards or people's opinions.

What part does your hair play in your life today? What in your "hair story" helped shape that?

I learnt that I had to sow to reap the rewards. I learnt that I had to look after my hair to see the rewards of healthy hair. But I didn't know what healthy hair was, which took some experimenting. I had to learn having a clean scalp didn't necessarily mean I had healthy hair, I had to learn about my curl pattern, moisturising, hot oil treatments, stretching, heat protection etc. I had to search for this information and ask lots of questions.

Luckily now, we have Afro hair social media influencers and Youtubers who share information and keep us informed. However, I had to learn that what works for them won't necessarily work for me. It was trial and error.

What more do you think needs to be done to empower Black women, particularly regarding hair and beauty?

Let people know that embracing your hair is also self-love. We need to be seeking out information and trying little things, like oiling your scalp, or a little head massage when you have a few minutes – it's all self-love.

Also, pay attention to the things we say to our children, which they subconsciously absorb. If, when growing up, a child constantly hears their parents moaning about their child's hair, calling it tough, hard to manage etc., then the child will take this on mentally and grow up constantly feeling those negative things about their hair.

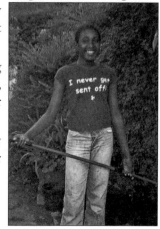

We have to foster that love from a young age, spend time giving children head massages, showing them how to moisture the ends of their hair or how to oil their scalp.

As Tyra Banks once said, "Self-love has very little to do with how you feel about your outer self. It's about accepting all of yourself."

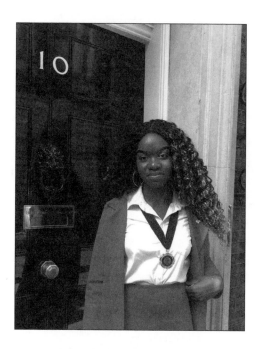

ANITA OKUNDE

Anita Okunde was born in Rochdale and is studying for her A Levels. She is a public speaker and activist for climate change. She hopes to go into politics and is a former member of the Youth Parliament, Greater Manchester's Youth Combined Authority and is involved in student leadership. By the age of 16, she had been to Downing Street twice, championing change on youth violence, particularly knife crime.

Anita has an enthusiastic approach, giving talks and appearing as a guest on panels, such as taking part recently in a discussion about animal welfare at the book launch for *Humane* by Polly Creed. She is the founder and president of Girl Up Manchester, and is an ambassador for Upendo Charity Organization.

What was your go-to hairstyle as a child, and who used to do your hair?

My go to hairstyle as a child was definitely a braided or cornrowed look! My mother is particularly good at hair and handled my hair as a child for the most part, but there was also a salon I went to sometimes if my mum didn't have the time as these hairstyles took many hours so it was nice to be able to experiment with different colours and styles!

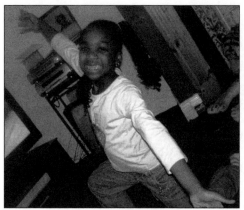

Who was your hair inspiration growing up?

I don't think I had a particular hair inspiration. The versatility of my hair meant I could do whatever I wanted and I think that was part of the magic for me. But once I entered my early teens the magic faded and I definitely held on to my relaxed hair to fit in with the Eurocentric view of beauty, which Afro texture hair didn't fit into. Now, I would say I'm still growing up but when I think of my Afro I think of the likes of Angela Davis, and the Black influencers I follow. There is a massive erasure of Afro-textured hair in the history books that needs to be brought to attention!

Who are the Black female role models in society, and how do they differ from the role models you had growing up?

I like the writer Jacqueline Wilson because I was a big reader and Malala Yousafzai, but they were never beauty based. They were my role models because they did amazing things or are important to my life which I think is something I'm happy I grasped as a child. With the amount of negative media about my hair, having role models that were beauty based would've probably ruined me. I don't think they have changed much in the sense of who I think of as my role models today but now I admire people like Angela Davis, Chimamanda Ngozi Adichie, still amazing people, just a different range, I guess. My role models now definitely have a lot more diversity and they look like me and they share so many interests with me which I think is really important because seeing myself in my role models is nice.

When you were younger, what beauty standards did you associate with being beautiful, and how do they differ today?

I definitely had a fixation on straight and long hair or looser curls, which was a lot different in comparison to my thick 4C hair. I was relaxed for most of my childhood too so I guess having those beauty standards imposed on my natural hair with the misconception that straight hair was easier to manage didn't help. However, now I'm a big "beauty is in the eye of the beholder" believer, and I have learnt to find beauty in everything which allows me to love myself and my hair a lot more and not have a set of beauty standards that upset me.

At what age were you made to feel like your hair was different? Tell us about that experience, what it felt like and how you navigated that?

This is a weird one because my hair was relaxed at a really young age so I grew up with technically "straight" hair. However, about three years ago now, I did the big chop and went fully natural which I guess was my navigation around my relationship with my hair and what it had to do with my self-worth. I used to use the excuse that relaxed hair was easier to maintain, instead of checking my ignorance around natural hair and definitely learning and making that decision to transition was a big step for me and I'm loving the journey!

What age were you when you started to make your own hair decisions, what were those decisions, and why did you choose the style you did?

I was about 12 when I started making my own hair decisions. I mean they weren't big decisions – it was more like, what hairstyles I would get to do for school and what colour they would be. That was quite limited because schools want all-natural hair colours but it was a very interesting journey because at that time my hair was still relaxed. I think my biggest decision was going natural and doing the big chop which is really cool when it comes to styles. I was always a big braids fan; they're really easy to have in and easy to maintain. You can wake up and your hair looks nice to go, so they were an easy one for me and my little thing was having my hair a bit curled at the end

Do you have any experiences where your hair had a major effect on something in your life?

Although my hair is really important to me and has a big role in my identity I don't think it has ever had a major effect on something in my life. It may have been a factor but not like the main cause of any problems. There was one time at school when I had to take my hairstyle out because it was too big and I think that was the angriest I've ever been about my hair. I had some long Afro-textured extensions which were really big and the school wasn't happy about them at all.

What part does your hair play in your life today? What in your "hair story" helped shape that?

I think I'm so much more comfortable with my hair now which has made it play a larger role in my life than it used to. I think that is great because I know right now there are a lot of people who look up to me. I think being able to show my natural hair and display it in a way that I feel comfortable with, which may not exactly be the usual media portrayal of natural hair, is really cool. Knowing that there are people who look at that and think maybe I don't have to have my natural hair slicked back or it doesn't have to be really loose curls, that is important to me because I like to think of myself as someone that people can look up to and be comfortable with. Showing my natural hair and my journey with it, is part of that.

What do you think about how brands situate themselves in the narrative of Black hair? What more do you think could be done?

I think the media can do so much more when we're looking at natural hair on Black women because what we tend to see is the slick backed high puffs with a lot of gel and product or 4A or 4B curls that are in a nicely set Afro and that's not what it looks like most of the time. We don't tend to see coverage of 4C curls or looking at hair that doesn't fit the stereotype that we've been given and that is so unhealthy especially for young Black girls growing up trying to navigate their hair journey because it makes them feel like their hair isn't worthy of the media or the front page covers. Whereas I think brands need to do better in making products that cater to curly and thicker hair and making sure that when they're running their adverts, they include women with curly hair and thicker hair and ensuring that they aren't being tokenistic about it. One model with loose curls set in an Afro isn't enough to show how diverse and versatile our hair is.

What do you think of the differences between the way Black men and Black women are treated in society when it comes to standards of beauty?

I don't think there are many differences when we are looking at the surface of it. Both have their hair seen as disorganized, or as unprofessional, which isn't ok, but it is the way it tends to be for Black men and women. However, I would say in the past few years Black men's hair has been more idolized and fetishized, especially by non-Black people. It's cool to have waves or dreads or braids for men and I think it's very interesting because Black women's hair hasn't been appreciated in the same way. I mean there's been appropriation for as long as I can remember but when it comes to the natural hair growing out of our heads, I still think it's disregarded as ugly and undesirable in a way that Black men's hair isn't, which is just an observation I've made.

What more do you think needs to be done to empower Black women, particularly regarding hair and beauty?

Well as the UK, artist ENNY said "These Black girls need to be on the shows." Media portrayal of Black women and their hair and beauty is very important when looking at empowering Black women. It's also really important to ensure that we are giving credit where credit is due for new styles, fashion, beauty and hair, which hasn't been done in the past few decades. Credit has been taken by other demographics of people when these ideas have originated with Black women, which is really sad, but it's something that's very apparent. I think if you want to grow past that and empower Black women, then they need to know that a lot of the trends and hairstyles that are seen as cool, or edgy on white women were theirs first.

What advice would you give to your younger self today? Or, what do you wish your younger self had known, that you know today?

The woman you become is going to meet and find many amazing Black women who rock their natural hair loud and proud. I hope that you find them soon too.

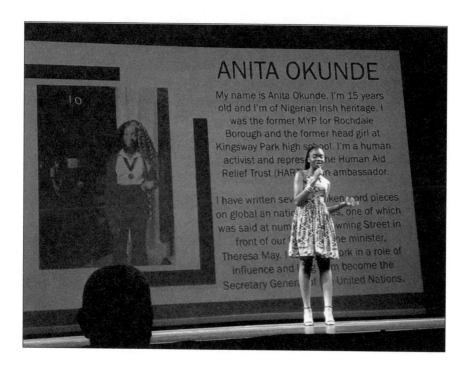

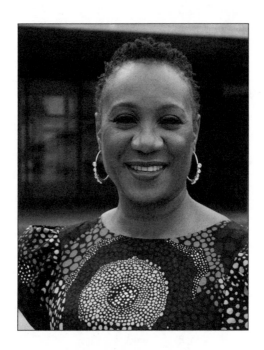

STELLA ONI

British Nigerian, Stella Oni, has a degree in Linguistics and African Languages from the University of Benin and a MSc in Information Systems and Technology from City University, London. She works as a Business Intelligence Analyst.

Stella is a cake enthusiast and an avid foodie who writes about Food, Culture and Tech on her blog African Britishness and the platform Medium. Her dream is to travel around the world to taste and experience food from different cultures. Stella believes that her experience of growing within two worlds has given her a unique perspective.

Her novel *Deadly Sacrifice* was shortlisted for the SI Leeds Literary Prize in 2016. It was published by Jacaranda Books in September 2020 and was Audible's Crime & Thriller pick of the month.

What was your go-to hairstyle as a child, and who used to do your hair?

My parents lived in England so I was with my grandmother in Lagos and Ibadan in Nigeria till the age of nine and remembered my hair going through many incarnations depending on my grandmother's exasperation and impatience.

The go-to was the traditional cornrows done by hulking women, that we called 'Mama onidiri' (Mama who plaits hair). I hated going to them because of their tendency to push your head into their ample laps to ensure they got the back of the head. I leave the rest to your imagination. Grandma would get fed up of my reluctance and so off to the barbers for a low hair cut. My grandma would periodically send photos of us to my parents in England and one time the barber had enthusiastically gone to town with my hair and left me with hardly any hair. I cried in horror so grandma decided to do the next best thing and that was to place a wig on my head, dress me in my best and take the photos. My mum was massively upset and I'm sure it was one of the reasons they decided it was time to come back to Nigeria and take over our care. May Grandma's soul rest in perfect peace.

Who was your hair inspiration growing up? Did you struggle to find Black hair inspiration?

Mariam Makeba for one. I am also a child of the 70s and 80s who fell in love with the African American Afros and Soul Train. We loved Kool and the Gang, The Jacksons, Chaka Khan, Whitney Houston and many others. It was so cool!

Who are the Black female role models in society, and how do they differ from the role models you had growing up?

The Black female role models for me now are Viola Davis, Angela Bassett and the writers. I loved Toni Morrisson and Maya Angelou. Growing up, I was more in love with the Black singers like Diana Ross, Chaka Khan, Whitney Houston. They exuded beauty, grace and massive unattainable talent.

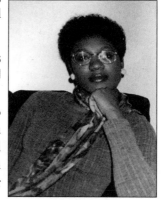

When you were young, what beauty standards did you associate with being beautiful, and how do they differ today?

Colourism is a big issue in Nigeria and it was no different when I was growing up. The lighter you are, the more desirable. I fell in between that and was fine. Conversely, girls that had deep dark skin were also admired but not as much as the lighter coloured ones. The standard of beauty today is more superficial and scarier. Young girls do not hesitate to go under the knife to augment various parts of their body.

At what age were you made to feel like your hair was different? Tell us about that experience, what it felt like and how you navigated that?

I grew up in Nigeria and so never felt my hair was different. What I wished for more than anything was for my hair to be thick and full. I had light hair but learnt to manage it. I had a curly perm from my university years to my early 30s and always had it professionally cut by a hairdresser.

What age were you when you started to make your own hair decisions, what were those decisions, and why did you choose the style you did?

I decided to spend more money making my hair beautiful. That meant regular trips to the hair salon for a curly perm and a sculpted hair cut. From my mid-thirties I began to use hair extensions, long plaits etc. I thought it made me look more sophisticated. I started to grow and groom my own natural hair about a year and half ago. The hair extensions and long plaits caused long term damage to my hairline. It is slowly growing back but it has taken years and an acceptance of my natural hair to have a healthy growth.

Do you have any experiences where your hair had a major effect on something in your life?

This is somewhat sad but natural hair was not as popular in the corporate world as it is now. I had hair extensions and wigs for many years and only recently had the confidence, after persuasion from a friend, to have my own hair. I love it now and will only occasionally wear a wig.

What part does your hair play in your life today? What in your "hair story" helped shape that?

Hair for me is freedom. I look in the mirror and I see the real me. I also have the choice to wear a wig if I like. My hair, my body.

What do you think about how brands situate themselves in the narrative of Black hair? What more do you think could be done?

The hair industry that serves Black hair is a billion pound one and not many companies are owned by Black people. That is very sad. The money flows out of the community but does not flow back. I think more and more Black people have started making products that are specifically for Black hair and people are consciously buying those products. It is slow because these are small businesses but I know it will grow into an industry one day.

What do you think of the differences between the way Black men and Black women are treated in society when it comes to standards of beauty?

Black men like to groom their hair in different ways but there are no pressures. Young Black women feel under pressure to conform to standards of beauty displayed on social media. That is unnatural.

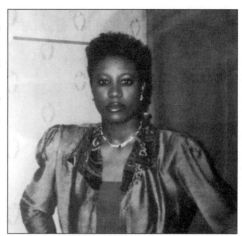

What more do you think needs to be done to empower Black women, particularly regarding hair and beauty?

The celebrities and influencers need to accept themselves because they have the power to influence the younger generation. Where they go, the rest will follow. At the moment, beauty is still aspiring to the light-skinned and hair extension or wigs, plus cosmetics. But the tide is turning slowly.

What advice would you give to your younger self today? Or, what do you wish your younger self had known, that you know today?

Girls suffer from different body image issues. I was no different. I was tall and thin in a society were being curvy and voluptuous was venerated. I grew into my body and I am still quite trim. I suffered terribly from feeling too thin, hair too scanty, legs too thin and that was from teasings over the years. I would have told myself to be confident and stand up for who I am.

Anything else you'd like to add?

Every trend comes and goes. It is important to continue to be true to ourselves and who we are. It took a long time for many of us to recognize that our strength lay in who we are and not how the world wanted us to be.

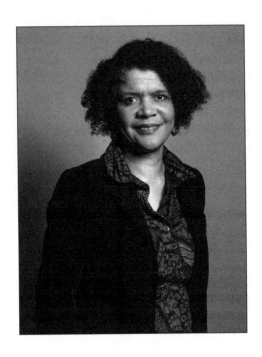

CHI ONWURAH

Chi Onwurah is a British Member of Parliament representing Newcastle upon Tyne Central and is also Shadow Minister Digital, Science & Technology. From 2016 – 2020 Chi was Shadow Minister for Industrial Strategy Science & Innovation (and Shadow Digital Minister Feb–April 2020). She has also held posts as Shadow Minister for Culture and the Digital Economy, Shadow Cabinet Office Minister leading on cyber security, social entrepreneurship, civil contingency, open government and transparency, Shadow Minister for Innovation, Science & Digital Infrastructure, working closely with the Science and business community, with industry on Broadband issues, and on the Enterprise and Regulatory Reform Bill.

Prior to Chi's election to Parliament in May 2010 she worked as Head of Telecom's Technology at the UK regulator Ofcom focussing on the implications for competition and regulation of the services and technologies associated with Next Generation Networks.

Prior to Ofcom, Chi was a Partner in Hammatan Ventures, a US technology consultancy, developing the GSM markets in Nigeria and South Africa.

Previously she was Director of Market Development with Teligent, a Global Wireless Local Loop operator and Director of Product Strategy at GTS. She has also worked for Cable & Wireless and Nortel as an engineer, project and product manager in the UK and France.

Chi is a Chartered Engineer with a BEng in Electrical Engineering from Imperial College London and an MBA from Manchester Business School. She was born in Wallsend and attended Kenton Comprehensive School in Newcastle, where she was elected the school's 'MP' in mock elections aged 17.

Chi is a Presidency Member of the Party of European Socialists (PES), and a Fellow of both the Institution of Engineering & Technology (FIET) and the City & Guilds of London Institute (FCGI) and also an Honorary Fellow of the British Science Assocation.

What was your go-to hairstyle when you were a child?

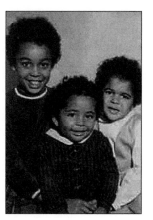

It was as an Afro. It was just what was washed and left to dry.

Who was your Black hair inspiration growing up?

I didn't have any. Diana Ross had fantastic hair. I used to love her hair and I used to sing her songs but I wasn't inspired by her hair. She was one of the only Black women who were visible back then.

Who are the Black female role models in society, and how do they differ from the role models you had growing up?

I think my mum was a role model for me. You're probably not going to have heard of some of the others. Now, there are women like Marie Emma McFadden; a Black British mathematician; Maggie Aderin Pocock, an astronomer and astrophysicist; the American politician Stacey Abrams, who fought against voter suppression in Georgia. There's also the IMF Director General Ngozi Okonjo-Iweala.

If there is one African American woman who inspired me when I was a child that would have to be Maya Angelou – and also bell hooks. She's certainly my political inspiration for my female transformation.

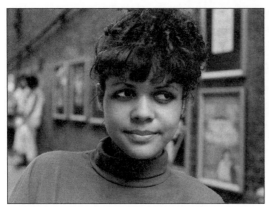

When you were young, what beauty standards did you associate with being beautiful, and how do they differ today?

It would have been from magazines like *Vogue*, and so it was very much a white, European standard of beauty. Whereas, what is great now is that there are many more African and African heritage standards of beauty, which I think is really liberating for someone like me.

At what age were you made to feel like your hair was different? Tell us about that experience, what it felt like and how you navigated that?

I mean, I would have been like, sort of five or six in primary school, and all my friends would be patting each other's hair. I mean, that's what I remember at school. But I knew that I was different from them, being the only Black person in the school from a very young age.

What age were you when you started to make your own hair decisions?

I was probably about 13 or 14. I don't remember really feeling that there were any choices. Also not having any money, I'd just get my hair cut by the local hairdressers, best they could. In Newcastle there were no places that were specifically for Black hair that I knew of.

Do you have any experiences where your hair had a major effect on something in your life?

I'm not sure. I mean, it's obviously hugely time-consuming at times, depending on what styles are in. Having my hair straightened in Paris I got my scalp burned once so that was impractical.

What do you think about how brands situate themselves in the narrative of Black hair? What more do you think could be done?

I think many brands are either confused or kind of patronizing. I launched the Black Beauty and Fashion Awards in 2017 which promotes equality and celebrates diverse beauty. Too many brands are fuelling racial stereotypes by lightening models' faces and not treating natural Black hair as normal. In developing countries, supposedly reputable cosmetic firms maximize their profits by claiming to make their customers whiter.

What do you think of the differences between the way Black men and Black women are treated in society when it comes to standards of beauty?

Black women have complicated standards to deal with but there are ways in which Black men are seen as being aggressive, which are related to standards of appearance and beauty, which define men as well. I think both Black men and women get stereotyped in ways which are really difficult to address.

What more do you think needs to be done to empower Black women, particularly regarding hair and beauty?

I think the growth of Black women wearing their natural hair, the whole sort of range of unprocessed styles, is really empowering. It means that girls should feel that they have choices that I never had growing up. I do think that magazines and cosmetics companies need to question the kinds of assumptions which underlie the imagery they use to sell their products. The brands that sell skin-lightening creams, should certainly be boycotted. They shouldn't be given any shelf-space.

Newspaper journalists need to be more knowledgeable too. I remember reading in *The Guardian* that Michelle Obama had chosen to have a short bob hairstyle for when Obama was campaigning – it being the easiest hairstyle to maintain. I think any Black woman knows that short, straight bobs are probably the hardest hairstyle to maintain.

I also think that Black hair is something that women, particularly Black women, bond through. I'd say that in Parliament, for example, where we have many Black female MPs, we all have different mixed appearances and we get trolled online. Obviously, Dianne Abbott, as the first Black woman MP, had to deal with a huge amount of prejudice in Parliament and still does on social media. I don't know how she's managed to weather it for so many years. She must just be able to ignore it somehow, or she doesn't read it. But she spoke really powerfully in Parliament recently about the impact of the online abuse on her staff, how it's hugely detrimental to their mental health.

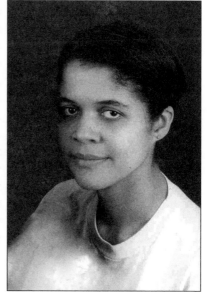

What advice would you give your younger self today?

Not to straighten my hair and to be confident with whatever way I look as an individual rather than trying to look like anyone else.

Anything you'd like to add?

Before I decided to wear my curly hair loose in the House of Commons, I had concerns about being seen as unprofessional. I wanted to be there representing Newcastle, my constituency, and I didn't want my constituents thinking that I wasn't paying enough attention to how I looked as an MP, for example, to do with dressing smartly and wearing my hair neat. So just a few days after I'd started wearing my hair natural and down this Black woman approached me on Westminster platform; she didn't know who I was. But she said, "I always like to congratulate Black women who have their hair natural, because I think that's an inspiration for other Black women. When I was young, I had to decide how I should be presenting myself so I often think back to that and I like to compliment Black women on their hair now."

I just think that was really nice and we need to do more of that.

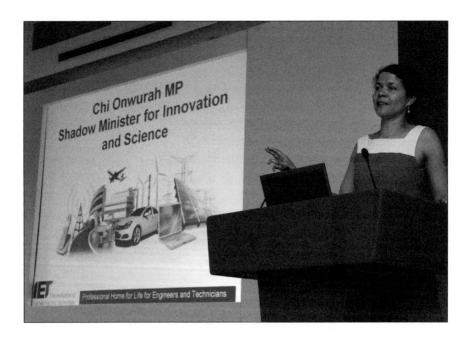

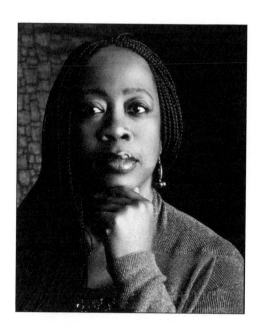

OLUSOLA OYELEYE

Olusola Oyeleye is an award-winning writer, director, dramaturg and producer working in opera, music theatre, visual arts, film, dance and education. She is a Senior lecturer in Acting at a faith-based university and is passionate about working with emerging creatives in community and educational settings.

Sola studied Physical Theatre at L'École Internationale de Théâtre Jacques Lecoq in Paris, and holds an MA in Contemporary Theatre Practice and Psychology from the University of Essex. She will start her doctoral studies next year. She was the first Black director to work at English National Opera and she set up Ariya, Britain's first Black opera company in 1994. Education, social justice and creativity run in her family. Her mother, a teacher and a nurse, regaled the family with real-life stories performed with an uncanny ability to mimic voices. Her father, a lawyer, spoke several languages, which became a passion in understanding that the key to a culture is through the power of communication. The ability to experience life as part of the Global Majority is a gift. She loves her name and is proud of her rich Yoruba cultural heritage.

Sola uses Drama to collaborate with organisations supporting victims of modern slavery, looked-after children and to encourage university access for disengaged youth. She says: "My Art is inextricably linked to my Faith, which is the engine of my creativity."

What was your go-to hairstyle as a child, and who used to do your hair?

When I was a baby I had a cute little Afro. As a toddler, my hair was long and very thick, so my mother plaited my hair with a central parting. Until today my hair naturally splits right down the middle. I don't need a comb, I can part it with my fingers. In my teens, when I wanted to have an Afro like Michael Jackson, that central parting was a big problem because it would just flop to the sides like a collapsing pack of cards. My mother put my hair in string plaits, which is a traditional West African style. I loved/hated sitting on the floor, cushioned between my mother's thighs, as she twisted the special thread around tufts of hair. The problem is, that I didn't really like anyone touching my head, so it was always a bit of a struggle. Pain-free, filled with intermittent conversation and wriggly movement. My mother would say that she, "couldn't wait until I could do my hair by myself." I thought my mother had the patience of a saint! Some years later, she admitted that she had behaved the same way with her own mother. My grandmother had said the same thing to her in Yoruba: "nko ni duro igbati ole şe irun rę funrararę". We both prefer to do our hair ourselves, and even today, when we enjoy those treasured moments of taking out, washing and redoing plaits, we still behave the same way, 'ouching' at moments that warrant a gentle touch. Most importantly, we laugh about it because we know how precious these moments really are. I am extremely grateful that we are so close.

Who was your hair inspiration growing up? Did you struggle to find Black hair inspiration?

I recognize now that I was in a cultural bubble growing up. There was school and home. Home was food, culture, music, language, art and politics. Although in primary school you could count the few children of African, Caribbean and Asian descent, we didn't have the language to navigate the 'colour prejudice'.

After my father passed away, following a short illness, we went to a more diverse school, where my sister and I were bullied by Caribbean and white students for being African, and for our 'primitive' hairstyles. I think this made me more determined to enjoy my natural hair in all its glory and to be proud of my cultural heritage. Home was a refuge from the storm. We were only four Black girls in my class at grammar school. One girl not only looked like Michael Jackson, but had the sweetest Afro. I really coveted that hairstyle. I loved traditional African hairstyles and was drawn to Angela Davis, Miriam Makeba, and my mother. With a lawyer and a teacher for parents, politics, social justice and education were rich threads of discussions and debates in the household. We were not always seen or heard, but we were certainly listening.

My mother occasionally hot combed my hair when I was a bridesmaid or for special parties. I have never, and will never, chemically straighten my hair. It has been challenging sometimes because of the way our society depicts beauty, but I can really be proud of myself that my hair is natural. On the occasions that I go to the hairdressers they always remark on my 'virgin' hair.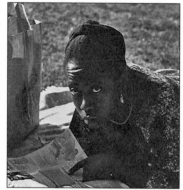

As a young adult, I would go to people's houses to get my hair plaited in singles with beads on the end. Honestly, a few whacks in the face from turning your head suddenly, could not discourage me from the joy of the wooden or glass beaded styles. That was until Bo Derek in *10*. All of a sudden beading hair was not an ancient tradition, but seemed to originate in a film with a woman running in slo-mo across a beach. Appropriation is real, dangerous and undermining. By all means enjoy, copy, but acknowledge and celebrate origins; but that's another story.

Who are the Black female role models in society, and how do they differ from the role models you had growing up?

One of the many joys of celebrating my African heritage is to be surrounded with culture and fashion in all its manifestions. So my hair role models appeared every time I stepped off the plane into the sauna of suffocating hot air at Murtala Muhammed International Airport. I celebrate my female relatives where culture and belief intertwine: Christian, Muslim and Fulani cultures all elicit spectacular hairstyles, not just for occasions, but for everyday life.

Looking back, I realize that I understood that hair was political with a capital 'P'. On film sets, there would be insensitive discussions about what they would do with my hair, and my actor colleagues would talk about their hair burning disasters, yet continue to perm. It cost a lot of money, and quite frankly, I decided to spend my money on life experiences and travel. There were clear sides: to be natural or to straighten. Doing your hair was not only a personal act, but a political one too. The lines are less clearly defined today. It is so interesting to see girls of every ethnicity wearing cane/cornrows.

When you were young, what beauty standards did you associate with being beautiful, and how do they differ today?

My parents limited what we watched on television. *Batman* and *Star Trek* were favourites, but we had a nurturing cultural ethos in the home. I was so used

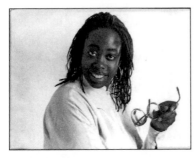

to my mother plaiting my hair, either on a Saturday ready for church, or on a Sunday afternoon, ready for school. It was rarely a weekday activity. My hair was always with a middle parting with two, four or eight connected plaits with the ends plaited together to make a neat loop. Occasionally, there might be a clip or hair pin. Our hairstyles were practical, made to last the week, the edges brushed each morning and the partings oiled midweek with Vaseline or Morgan's pomade or Sulfur 8 for the healthy shine. As a child, my she-roes were Lieutenent Uhura on *Star Trek* and Eartha Kitt as Catwoman. Everything about Catwoman was 'purrfect'! Her hairstyle was easily accessible by twisting my fingers through my hair to make curls. My fingers were my natural rollers. I would make a fringe by twisting my hair around one finger and using the next to hold it together like a clip. It was very satisfying to see the effect. With natural hair, even when hot combed, the finger curls would only last a day or two. As a teenager I kept the same simple natural styles. As my hair was quite long and thick, I loved twisting my hair, pulling it back into a small bun, and then after a week untwisting each plait to make a frenzy of curls. These were some of my favourite hair styles. I think partly I enjoyed the volume of having big hair, and also because I had complete control over how I dressed my hair. It always feels very empowering, even today. I particularly liked that fact that you could never be quite sure how it would turn out!

I had always wanted to buy a wig, but I never had the courage, until a couple of years ago when I met up with one of my former students who took me to a hair shop. We spent a wonderful hour trying on wigs and I bought one, a short bob. I have only worn it once. I should have bought hair pins because I had to keep pulling it forward as I could feel it gently slipping back and the fringe which was just above my eyebrows began to look like Julie Andrews in the *Sound of Music* or the lead in the film *Amelie*. I got lots of compliments, but I was forever conscious that I was wearing a 'hair hat'. There seemed to be a lot of pressure to conform to a standard of beauty that did not include or celebrate my cultural heritage and I instinctively fought against it.

Perming hair was expensive and I remember distinctly saying at 18, that I had better things to spend my money on. I celebrated hair plaiting, even though you had to put a whole day aside, while the hairdresser answered calls, fed her children, fed herself, went to the shops to buy something that she had forgotten... Once the hairdresser even got her children plaiting my hair shortly after they came back from school. They seemed content, encouraged by their mother talking to them in French about all the nice things they could buy with the money. Seriously, the conversations that take place when people are doing your hair, is a little like doctors doing their rounds and talking about the patient rather than to them. For the 4, 5, 6, 7, 8… 9 hours you are there, your head is dissociated from the rest of your body. All you are is a head! I have had some awful experiences at hairdressers so I rarely go to salons. Sadly, I have found that many Black hairdressers, particularly the younger ones, are used to working with chemically permed hair, so my 'virgin' hair has been pulled and tugged to oblivion. On one occasion, after washing my hair, the hairdresser left me and attended to others until my hair was almost dry, after some tugging and combing without holding the base: my painful protests brought an older woman over. She complimented me on my natural hair and blow-dried it so carefully that I felt beautiful once more.

Hair was intrinsically linked with the Black Power movement and it was sad to see so many women conflicted. I say let freedom reign. Today people can do what they like. There are some 'hairstyles' one would not be allowed to leave the house with. You know the ones that look like you just got out of bed, or you just unplaited your hair. I think it's great that many Black women do not care about conformity, they just do what they like, and I think that it is a cause for celebration.

At what age were you made to feel that your hair was different? Tell us about that experience, what it felt like and how you navigated that?

I always knew, but I was not in conflict with my hair, but my hair was often in conflict with me. Remember, I didn't really enjoy anyone touching my hair. Sometimes my hair decided not to co-operate with me. Punished me for no good reason. Admittedly, I know why. Sometimes, I would leave my plaits in too long. The ensuing operation to unpick, untangle, massage knots into freedom was always followed by promises to do better, until the next time. Everything was alright when my mother dressed my hair, but anyone else: problem. My mother held my hair tightly at the base. Secure and painless tugs of the comb were soothing, tolerated, necessary weekly activities. Painless. Anyone else seemed to forget the thick curls. The comb was like a machete crashing through a thicket of unruly bush, and only devastation ensued. Long thick, curly hair, washed and not oiled immediately, equals pain and headaches as the pick comb massacred the big impenetrable knots that were always hidden from view, but felt like your head was about to explode on first touch. Imagine a tangled ball of wool, where the knitter carefully tries to untangle the unruly mesh, then gives up, pulls and tugs to oblivion. Until recently, I never went to a salon because even some Black hairdressers seem to find natural hair challenging. If you cause me pain once, I will never go back. Fortunately, there are amazingly talented women and men who respect, cherish and celebrate all the hair textures that we have been blessed with. Amen to that!

What age were you when you started to make your own hair decisions, what were those decisions, and why did you choose the style you did?

The first time I got the, "Yes, you can go out with your own hairstyle" approval was aged 10 years old. Straight parting, very important, and two plaits equidistant with the ends plaited into a loop and tucked neatly into the base of one plait. It wasn't a different style, it was simply that my mother was relieved to be passing on the baton. A rite of passage. Any mother whose daughter is a whinger and moaner at hair washing and plaiting time will empathize. It was exciting to be free, to be able to say: "I can do it myself", and my mother had to accept that the time of the "Hair Wars" was finally over. It would be several years later, when I began to plait my own hair in singles, without extensions, and have the autonomy to schedule in the time to do my hair, that I was able to reflect on the precious time spent sat between my mother's knees 'ouching' and 'ouching' at the very occasional loosening of grip when combing out, that emitted an involuntary squeal of discomfort, that didn't hurt, but just reflected an inherited aversion to anyone doing my hair. I've grown out of it. I have learnt to endure.

Do you have any experiences where your hair had a major effect on something in your life?

That my hair has always been natural is a blessing and very empowering. The real challenge is staying true to myself, whilst enjoying the wonderful diversity of styles available. Even now, when I do crochet braids, my hair is neatly plaited in cornrows underneath and it is liberating. I feel a sense of personal pride that I did not succumb to all the different negative tropes, and stayed strong in celebrating the hair I was born with. There is a contradiction though, I love the way the millennials unplait-and-go. In my day, that would not have been accepted, those hairstyles are for home days. Now the bushier the better: curls, wigs, kinky, dreadlocks…anything goes.

I was recently licensed as a Lay Minister (LLM), a Reader in the Church of England. Our licensing was at Southwark Cathedral and we were very fortunate to have the service between the second and third lockdowns. I was considering wearing a headwrap, but in the end, decided to wear my hair in crochet braids. The decision was personal, without conflict, but it was interesting for me to reflect on why I made that decision for the ceremony. Everything is political, even the air we breathe.

How do you wear your hair at work? Or for interviews? Has this changed over time?

For most of my adult life, I have worn head-wraps. Both as an acknowledgement of my

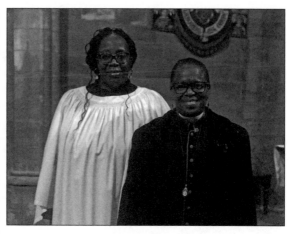

African heritage, but also for those bad hair days, and I've had many of those. Even on those days, I am secure in the knowledge that whatever condition my hair is in, it's mine, and I love my hair. The other reason relates to people wanting to touch my hair. I work in the Arts, and I am also an academic: there is quite a lot of individuality in those arenas. But honestly, the fascination with Black hair still catches me off-guard. Even rare specimens or exhibits in a museum or art gallery get handled more carefully. The reverence and wonder are not welcome, and I still don't think people understand why. New hairstyles will draw hand-phantoms that reach out from unknown places to touch, tug, pull, fluff, comment with fascination on whatever hairstyle appears that week or day. Compliments all appreciated. I am tolerant, but please don't touch my hair. I don't know where your hands have been! Honestly, I have to laugh. Remember when people got a wind that Black women were using extensions, and it was juju that our hair changed length or curl or colour from time to time? When asked if my hair is mine, I love the old adage, "It's mine, I bought it!" Work colleagues have mentioned that they haven't seen my hair, but love my colourful headwraps. Occasionally, I gave them a hair treat. Headwraps off, hairstyle out, particularly in the summer heat. Winter comes, headwraps on.

What part does your hair play in your life today? What in your "hair story" helped shape that?

My choice to stay natural has had a profound effect on my sense of self. It has taught me to stand up for what I believe in, while embracing diversity of choice. Hair is not a binary discussion. The complexity of thought, tradition and discourse is real. Our choices are our own. I am encouraged by the cross-cultural nature of hairstyles and traditions, but we still need to acknowledge

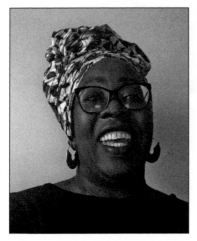

the historical context of styles and not denude them as just fashions or trends.

What do you think about how brands situate themselves in the narrative of Black hair? What more do you think could be done?

There are fewer Black-owned hair businesses in the UK. It feels very different in continental Europe and in the US, where Black-owned hair businesses have a greater share of the market. Our cultures have been appropriated for centuries without respectful acknowledgement, and even when acknowledgment is given, it is given begrudgingly.

Personally, I choose very simple hair products: baby shampoo and conditioner and a wash-in product I discovered recently for special occasions. Olive, coconut and castor oil with ginger. Even Vaseline still gets a look in. I feel vindicated for not giving into the pressure perm. Everything has turned full circle, and I get to enjoy everything that is available. I still want to get another wig!

What do you think of beauty products such as skin-lightening creams?

Shadism is so prevalent cross-culturally; a legacy of slavery, indentured labour and caste systems. As long as societies sit in the post-colonial state of psychological dysfunction, and definitions of beauty are so narrow, then the non-medical skin-lightening industry will continue to thrive. Black is beautiful. Let us hope that those people who use those creams will be comfortable within themselves, and have the strength mentally and physically to combat the negative and destructive signalling around depth or lightness of skin colour. Frantz Fanon's analysis of colonization and the processes of decolonization should be essential reading for everyone. I take inspiration from the Ghanaian Adinkra symbol Sankofa: "We must understand the past to look forward to the future."

Can you easily find beauty products which suit your skin tone?

I rarely wear make-up, but I have enjoyed having the occasional makeover. I have learnt what suits me and I stick to it.

What do you think of the differences between the way Black men and Black women are treated in society when it comes to standards of beauty?

Men have gone through their own journey, which is as challenging and diverse as women's, all mixed with societal expectations, tropes and imagery. There is definitely a long story there. I have brothers, so I know it is complex.

What more do you think needs to be done to empower Black women, particulary regarding hair and beauty?

One of the formative experiences of my life was a research trip to Lagos to meet the great Nigerian phototographer J.D. Okhai Ojeikere who spent a lifetime photographing the traditional hairstyles of Nigerian women with their names and meanings. His wonderful photographic archive and books are a celebration of the artistry of hair and string plaiting. A reminder that hair fashion is deeply-rooted in culture: symbolic and powerful. It speaks of ancestry, community past, present and future. Looking at his work, I am inspired to start string plaiting my hair again.

What advice would you give to your younger self today? Or, what do you wish your younger self had known, that you know today?

Navigating notions of beauty is hard, even when you have good role models. Their love sustains you, but they can't follow you into toxic unwelcoming spaces. They can only be the wisdom you receive, the refuge of comfort and the balm to heal the arrows. I believed deeply that I wasn't going to use chemicals to straighten my hair. I don't like the feeling of being coerced into something that meant, at that time, that I had to 'deny' myself to 'gain' an acceptable version of myself. For the times when I felt pretty, but was not treated as such and the times when the comments about how much more attractive I could look were related to 'straight' or 'curl'. For the days when I literally laughed and cried about my hair, I applaud my younger self, through the grace and wisdom of my mother, for setting the example to have the courage to love and be myself. Amen to that!

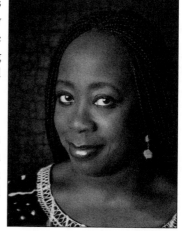

Anything else you'd like to add?

I have the right to define my own hair. It's mine. My hair is not a number or a letter from the alphabet. My hair is just protein and skin cells: but my hair, my African curly, natural hair is awesome.

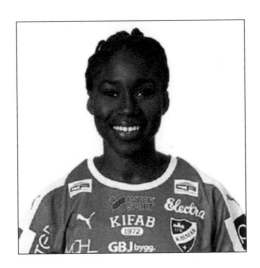

SHADE PRATT

Folashade Pratt is an athlete and footwear design apprentice at Nike.

Pratt attended the Rosemount High School at her hometown. In her time there she earned several accolades, including being nominated two-times All-Metro selection, two-times all-state and three-times all-conference selection. In 2011 Pratt went to University of Maryland. She played only seven matches in her freshman year. In her sophomore year, she became a starter for the Terrapins, playing mostly as a wide midfield and a wide back. In her junior year, Pratt played for the first time in her career as a centre-back. In her senior year, after several Terrapins were sidelined by injuries, Pratt was moved to frontline, becoming a forward. Pratt was the 25th overall pick in the 2015 NWSL College Draft when she was picked by Sky Blue FC. Pratt only played one match for the SBFC, on June 28, 2015 against Chicago Red Stars. For the 2016 National Women's Soccer League season, Pratt signed with Portland Thorns FC. She played five matches for the Thorns in that season.

In 2017 she was signed to the Norwegian top club Røa Dynamite Girls. From August she was on loan to another club in the same division, Stabæk Chixa. She signed with the Swedish club IFK Kalmar in January 2018. In June 2019 she signed with the Portuguese champions, Braga.

She is also a designer and artist.

What was your go-to hairstyle as a child, and who used to do your hair?

My go-to hairstyle was the four little braids with the barrettes at the bottom, and my mom used to do it. Classic.

Did you have any hair inspiration growing up, and if so, did you struggle to find Black female hair inspiration?

Growing up, I was in Maryland, which was more diverse, so I was around many races, so I think there was a lot of hair inspiration around me there. It wasn't until I moved to Minnesota, where I was then in the minority, that it became more difficult to find. That was when I was getting into my teen years. It bothered me more in high school, trying to fit in, being on sports teams, and I would be the only Black woman on my team, so then when it came to travelling and things, we couldn't share products and stuff because they didn't use anything I used. But it wasn't too bad.

You kind of find the community here and there, and hairstylists do your hair. I think as years went on more hairstylists started opening shops in the suburbs so we didn't have to go all the way down into the twin cities.

Who would you say are the Black female role models in society now, and how do they differ from the role models you had growing up?

I don't have any role models in particular, but I think a lot of Black women in society, from celebrities to whoever are our role models now, are embracing this natural hair journey, and you can literally see it on TV and at award shows. Even if you're straightening your hair no one is discouraging that, but everyone is accepting how you like to do your hair, and no one can take that away from you. Compared with when I was growing up, when we used to see the Dark and Lovely relaxer promoted, and you'd see all the stars straightening their hair, and it was this whole thing about trying to fit into society, be what we're not, and damaging our hair.

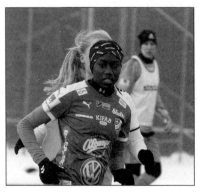

Now you see these young kids with luscious hair flowing with their Afros, and it's so cute to see everyone embracing their curls. And back in the day, it wasn't even that relaxers were advertised on TV, but you saw celebrities with long straight hair, and then you went into the hair salon and said, "I wanna look like them". In the hair salons, they were pushing the relaxers as well, or you would go to buy your products, and it's there. Now I can't even find a relaxer on the shelf. You'd go into a department store, and you'd see all of our products together, it used to be just the boxes. Now we have all the natural hair care products in one section, and this is much better.

When you were young, what beauty standards did you associate with being beautiful, and how do they differ today?

Straight blonde hair was the beauty standard. Today, I can't even be bothered. Black women's hair is the most universal hair there is. There's no other people like us with our hair. You can look across all the other races, and some people will have straight hair that falls, others will have curly hair, but no one has our kind of hair; we can do literally everything and anything possible with our hair.

I've always been of darker complexion so that was always a joke within middle school, because I arrived in Minnesota the summer before my fifth grade year. I'd never been around so many white people before. Maryland has some of the richest Black neighbourhoods in America, where you can also find diversity at every corner. Coming to Minnesota I was exposed to something I had never seen before. I was the token Black kid in class and people were just being curious and wanting to touch my hair and I was like, "No, don't mess up the poof!" My brother used to wear his hair in an Afro and it was nice and plush in the morning but by the end of the day it would be squashed.

What age were you when you started to make your own hair decisions?

I was really into crochet braids and stuff like that, but my parents were pretty chill so they would kind of let me do whatever, within restraint. I remember that it wasn't until I got to Minnesota that I was like, "Hey Mom, can I relax my hair?" and she'd tell me, "No, you're too young. When you get to a certain age, then maybe we can try." Looking back I understand that then it was the thing to do. Especially if you're playing sports with the way we wear our hair – everyone kind of wears it in a slicked-back ponytail but then you're sweating, so it isn't going to last very long. I was getting into sports heavily, and I was trying to fit in more.

Do you have any experiences where your hair had a major effect on something in your life?

The natural trend started to happen when I was in college. Thank god for me, I went to the University of Maryland, not because I was from there, just by coincidence. I played soccer and track, and the track team was a bit more diverse. Track athletes care about their hair. We don't just go out there. Some people do their make-up, and I had a couple of friends on the team who were really into hair, and that's when they started their natural hair journey. You'd see all over campus some people were doing the big chops and that was like, "Wow! We can do that?" Then there were people helping you, saying, "OK, these are the products I'm using." When you looked at people, it was like, "Wow! She chopped her hair a year ago and look at what it is now," so that was really inspiring for me.

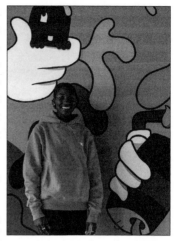

How do you wear your hair at work? Has this changed over time?

My work as a sports person is going to practice so I don't do anything special with my hair. I can come in a T shirt and sneakers. Now that I work in the art and design world, it's more about being yourself. You're accepted for you and there is usually no need to wear a suit and tie like in other places of employment.

Since you can be so free, have you ever done anything like pink braids?

No. I've never been a person who experimented too much with my hair. I've never done the big chop. I'll cut the dead ends maybe, but nothing too crazy. I get box braids sometimes, I just change up the length for different events.

What part does your hair play in your life today? What in your "hair story" helped shape that?

It gives you confidence when you get a new hairstyle. Seeing other people in college inspired me, and I would also say living abroad, in Norway. It was easier for me to embrace my natural hair over there because they had no idea what was going on. That was my way of getting a lot of the damage out that I'd done from overly straightening my hair and heat damage. That was when I started getting ideas of how I wanted to do my hair and developed a lot of the practices I use today. I don't own a blow-dryer anymore, it's very rare that I would ever blow-dry my hair. I also learned how to box braid my own hair. It wasn't good but I used YouTube and figured it out.

What do you think about how brands situate themselves in the narrative of Black hair? What more do you think could be done?

I think the majority of brands try to advertise that their product works for all and that's not always the case. Obviously, with influencers these days and people doing try-on videos, if the product is good, we will come together because it's for us. But we don't feel bad about not being included in something that is not for us; we don't need to be included there. I think everyone wants to include us in everything just so they can say that their product is diverse, even if it's not!

What do you think of the differences between the way Black men and Black women are treated in society when it comes to standards of beauty?

When it comes to standards of beauty, it seems often that Black women and men are left out of the conversation. For so long, there has been a European standard of beauty shoved down our throats. In terms of hair, Black women have endured a lot from being told how society thinks we should wear our hair to the grocery store, to work – you name it.

What more do you think needs to be done to empower Black women particularly in regards to hair and beauty?

I still think we need more representation. It's getting there but it's not enough. I don't see what's wrong with having a campaign featuring Black women. We're always the minority and it would be such a change if you saw mostly Black women in a hair campaign and one white woman. People would automatically think the campaign is for Black people but that's how things get presented to us in hair and beauty. It's usually all white women and one Black person or an Asian person. We're always the minority and I just think it needs to be more normalized that people are people and have these different faces which appear daily because we're in real life daily. So more representation.

If you could give any advice to your younger self, what would you say? Is there something you wish you had known when you were younger that you now know?

Probably, that, "You are beautiful and your hair is beautiful. Embrace who you are and every bit of your Blackness!"

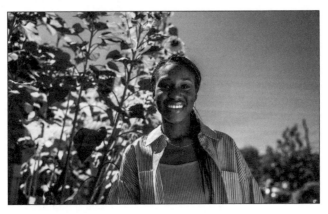

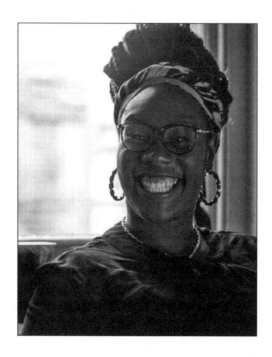

RIANNA RAYMOND-WILLIAMS

Rianna Raymond-Williams is the founder and managing director for Shine ALOUD UK, a social enterprise that uses creative media and peer-led training to empower young people and adults to talk about sexual health and relationships. She works as a sexual health advisor for the NHS in London, providing STI and HIV results to patients, safer sex messaging and behaviour change counselling, alongside referrals to third-party organisations, to support a range of patients to manage their health and well-being.

Rianna has a BA in Journalism from the University of Arts London and a Master's Degree in Reproductive and Sexual Health Research from the London School of Hygiene and Tropical Medicine. She is currently undertaking a PhD at Glasgow Caledonian University in London, where she will be exploring how Black women make sense of their sexual identity in the UK.

Rianna is also a journalist who covers sexual health and well-being, identity, race and digital media for *The Voice* Newspaper, *Black Ballad*, *The Independent*, gal-dem and SH:24.

What was your go-to hairstyle as a child, and who used to do your hair?

My go-to hairstyle was called 'cup and saucer'. My mum used to plait my hair into four or five plaits on the side and one in the middle. She did my hair up until the age of about nine or ten. Throughout my childhood, my mum wore her natural hair in a big Afro, it was thick, long and lovely, but then she started wearing extensions. As a child, I didn't understand why she was putting "extra" hair on her head, but I wanted to look like my mum, so I started to get hair extensions too. Then I went through a phase of doing my hair myself – I learned to cornrow my hair, I learned to do single plaits and sew-in weave. A lot of Black girls I went to school with – and I – used to walk around with our hair half out and half done. Half of our hair would be done - in braids, cornrow or slicked up with pink gel, and the other part of it wouldn't, but we'd find someone else at school to do it for us. This was a normal thing for us. We would all sit in the playground together; someone would be cornrowing, someone would be putting in beads, others were using the hard brush and gel to activate edges and finger waves – it was an experience!

Who was your hair inspiration growing up? Did you struggle to find Black hair inspiration?

Raven from *That's So Raven*. I think it's because she was another Black woman on TV. I remember buying a big Vidal Sassoon blow-dryer. I didn't know back then but her hair was clearly relaxed. So, I tried to use the blow dryer on my hair to get the same style, but it just began to break. I even went through a period of straighteners. I don't know why or how that happened, we just started straightening our hair at school. We had a salon enterprise in our school to encourage us to get some practical skills in hair and beauty. I think our teachers realized that we were doing each other's hair, so they thought, let's give them a place to do that. You could pay, say, 50p to come and do your hair, you could get a massage, get your nails done – it was really good, now I think about it. We were looking after each other – we were a group of predominantly young Black girls actively invested in the self-care of one other, which was a beautiful thing. Me and my best friend became salon managers! But as good as it was, I realize there were only particular people involved – young Black girls!

Who are the Black female role models in society, and how do they differ from the role models you had growing up?

Today, young girls look up to women like Nicki Minaj, Megan Thee Stallion, Cardi B. In the UK, Jorja Smith, Stefflon Don, Nao and Ella May. I think there's a sex element to it, particularly with US artists. A friend told me about a time she was working with some young girls at a school, and they had this thing called 'boss day' – it was an opportunity for all of these girls to come in and dress in the way they saw "bosses". She said all of these girls rolled up to the school looking like Nicki Minaj, because she is the boss that they see, but little did they know that people in the corporate sector who are bosses don't look like that. Some of them have loose-fitting clothing, no make-up, no jewellery. But their aspiration was this Black woman who looks really sexy, and obviously has loads of money and cars. So what we idealize is not always the truth. Entertainment is different from real life.

There are Black women in literature like Bernadine Evaristo and Reni Eddo-Lodge who are inspirational and successful. Both of these women don't over exaggerate their presentation – they're comfortable in themselves and they present in that way. I think people like and respect them, but their 'image' is too simple for some people to aspire to. It's sad because I think it then creates the idea that you have to look a particular way to be successful and if you don't, you're not successful. There's something to be said about putting on this mask to be accepted in particular spaces and circles. That comes with the hair you wear, the make-up, the nails you wear – or don't. Feeling like you need to have this thing to belong, otherwise you're an outcast. I think Black women feel that even more because of the intersections of identity: we're Black, we're women – and class has a part to play in how we are received too. Often, assumptions are made about our body and character, and if we live up to these stereotypes we are judged, and if we don't, we are judged too.

When you were young, what beauty standards did you associate with being beautiful, and how do they differ today?

Hair definitely was a big part of it… and size as well. There's always been this culture of fat-shaming, and I've always been a big person. But now we see shape is what everybody wants to have – just not on Black women. Everybody wants to have fuller lips, fuller figures, bums, breasts, but if you're Black it's a problem – it's offensive, even. I went to a school that was predominantly made up of Asian women and Black women, but you feel invisible in the media, you know there's nobody that looks like you, and when they do, they're always very unconventional or different and then you feel like, why should this person represent me? We should have variations of different people. Kevin and Perry from *Kevin and Perry Go Large* do not speak for all white men, white women or non-binary people, but Libby 'Squiggle' on *EastEnders*, is meant to speak for all Black women? If you're Black and in the media, you're forced to speak for everyone. I also think it's about projection. People want to keep this vision of us. Of Black men being big and dangerous, of Black women being hostile or

189

unfriendly. All of these personas that people have created about us that are not true creates a disconnect between us and our lived experiences.

I think we need to put these experiences in context and ask: why is this Black woman angry? Because she's walked into the shop to buy a product and she's being followed by a security guard who thinks she's a thief, or she can't find her shade of make-up. This says that she's visible as a criminal, but invisible to the beauty world. And if you experience things like this on a regular basis you're going to feel angry, you're going to feel frustrated, and people want to say you're angry for no reason. When I did an Erasmus exchange in my early teens I went to Bulgaria. I attended a youth conference and I was the only Black person there. There was a group of young people looking at me, staring and laughing. I asked their supervisor, "Why are they doing this?" He said, "They think you're beautiful, they have never seen a Black woman before." At that moment, I noticed they were deaf young people, but they used their hands and arms to ask me if I could swim, which I found really offensive. They looked at me as though I was not human. I remember feeling really insecure because I'd never experienced anything like it before. Living in London, which is really diverse, you forget how closed off the rest of the world is, and then you have experiences like that.

At what age were you made to feel like your hair was different? Tell us about that experience, what it felt like and how you navigated that?

I think I'd always known, but I had an experience in Year 9. In our school,

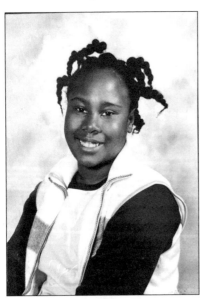

we used to walk around with our hair out a lot. I remember being in my English class and part of my hair was out, part of it was plaited – and my English teacher, who was an Indian-St Lucian woman with really long curly hair, said, "Rianna, why is your hair like that? It's very messy." I was confused and thought, this is how my hair grows out of my head! And you, as a Black woman, why would you say that to me? But there are elements of colourism that come into it, because her hair in its natural state grows downwards, whereas my hair in its natural state is out and loud. I also used to walk around with my hair fully out, and I remember my friends asking me, "Can I touch your

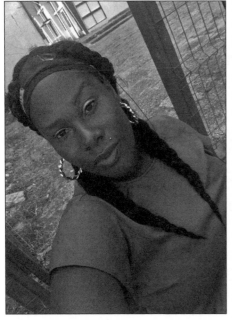

hair?" but I never knew why. And that made me think: maybe my hair is different. Even though my school was mostly a mix of Black and Asian ethnicities, I did think there were expectations of how Black girls should be. I used to hear: "You're not like the rest of the Black girls, you're really nice", and I used to think, what does that even mean? But I also know there's a lot of anti-Blackness in Asian communities, and they have their own issues with colourism. Their families may have said things about Black children – the typical stereotypes of: Black people steal; they're lazy. Maybe because I didn't fit that perception, having first-hand interactions with me in school made them think, "This doesn't fit what I've been told." Sometimes we don't even know we're being taught to believe these things. And it's terrible because then we're doing it to ourselves – distinguishing who is Black and who isn't Black enough by using words like coconut or Oreo to refer to our own people. People discriminate against us, and we pick this up and use this same discrimination towards each other as a kind of protection for ourselves to prove our own Blackness.

Do you have any experiences where your hair had a major effect on something in your life?

My mum had a bad experience with a hot comb when she was younger. My granny was doing her hair for her by the stove in the kitchen, and she turned around by accident and the hot comb went into her eye. They had to rush to the hospital. She was fine, but it just shows you the pain that we can and do go through for our hair. I know loads of other Black women who have stories of pain or trauma too when it comes to hair. My mum always used to rock an Afro to work, and then I think she said in a passing conversation: "They always want to put their hand in my hair", and, "Who do they think they are?" I don't think she had a language for these microaggressions back then. My mum now has beautiful long dreads which she's been growing for about 10 years or more now; she wanted to start the process a lot earlier, but even I didn't want her to have dreads because of what is typically associated with people who wear their hair in dreadlocks, which is terrible, but my young and immature mind knew nothing different from what the media was telling us about Rastafarians being dangerous and linked to criminality, which couldn't be further from the truth, but a clear indication of how racial stereotyping continues to create negative ideas about communities, that even the communities themselves begin to internalize them. Now I'm in the process of doing my hair in dreads!

I remember a friend who used to spend ridiculous money on wigs. She would say it was an investment. And I just didn't understand why she would spend so much money when she had lovely hair growing out of her head, but the truth is that many of us feed into this perception that says you're only beautiful if you have Peruvian, Brazilian or Moroccan hair coming out of your head. Which is totally not true. But as you grow and you learn, you develop a healthier sense of self-esteem, and better friendship circles and can be honest about these things. We don't typically see representations of Black women without fake hair on their heads. So unless you have these representations in your own family, or have grown up with them, you won't see them. I watched a lot of old films from the 60s and 70s starring Black people, and I'm always interested in the Black experience of the first generation who came here – to the UK. They had huge Afros and beautiful hair, and it looked so powerful. Nobody teaches us about our hair; the power of our hair, what hair means for us. And I'm not sure many of our parents or grandparents know either. I know very brief histories – I know cornrows helped to direct enslaved people to freedom – it's amazing, we are very creative people, but we're not in tune with that side of us enough. The other side of this is that Black women are able to make a business out of hair care. And at the time, my friend was buying from a friend who was making wigs on the side of an admin job, and I thought that was amazing – let her use her skills to make money for herself and make other women feel great too.

What part does your hair play in your life today and what in your hair story shaped that?

For me, my hair is very powerful, and it's part of my identity. Over the last two years, I've gone on my own journey where I started to loc it, but I wasn't sure, so I was combing parts of it out and some of it was still in locs, and I was like, what am I going to do? Growing up I always wanted to be a hairdresser, but I've got even less patience now than I had when I was younger, so that's not going to happen any time soon! But I think hair is so beautiful, particularly Black hair – because I used to do hair I could see how it could be transformed in terms of washing, drying, cornrowing, styling, and I think it's such a creative process. Your hair says a lot about you; how you manage it says a lot about your identity. My mum has impacted my own journey a lot. I have seen how beautiful and long my mum's hair is and I want the same for myself – I don't want to be burning my hair with dryers, and sowing and weaving, I just want to let my hair grow from my head naturally.

What do you think about how brands situate themselves in the narrative of Black hair? What more do you think could be done?

I was once in Sainsbury's – in the 'ethnic' aisle – and I told a worker that 'ethnic' is not the right term, and they just looked at me like I was crazy, but a couple of months later it was changed to 'World Foods'. Things like that show you how insensitive people are to other people's cultures. There's a lot to be said about visibility, and Black people have for a long time lived in the UK, but we can't find our products in particular shops – why is that? Why is it we can only find our products in a Black magazine or in Black hair shops? If you go into a Black hair shop you might see a Black magazine – why is that not in a general shop like a newsagents? I think there's a market that's being missed.

What do you think of the differences between the way Black men and Black women are treated in society when it comes to standards of beauty?

I was saying to my friend the other day: part of me feels like it's easier for some men – I would say, generally, that men can just show up in a T shirt and jeans. Whereas with women: if you're showing cleavage it's a problem; if you've got nails it's a problem; if you've got earrings it's a problem; if your hair's not right it's a problem. Even the clothes we want to wear – if you've got a fuller body it can be seen as more revealing. I wore leggings for a long time because they were comfortable, but I didn't think they were sexy, they were just clothes. But because my body is a particular way, people think I'm being revealing, or suggestive, but no: my body is just the way it is. Women have a harder time for sure. It's just another thing we have to deal with in the world.

What more do you think needs to be done to empower Black women, particularly regarding hair and beauty?

Visible representation: we need to see more Black women. We also need to have a conversation about what hair care looks like. Initially, when we started the salon in our school, there was a Black woman who started it with us, Ms George. I remember she spoke to us about coconut oil and how to wash our hair. Someone to actually sit down with Black women and teach them that their hair is part of them and not another thing to deal with is so important.

It's part of the whole therapeutic nature of looking after yourself and who you are, and your hair is a part of that. It should be part of our daily routine, and if it takes as long as it does, so be it. And being true about what we need as well – whether that's sleep or food, because all of that impacts how our hair grows, how our nails grow. We don't make enough time to think about all the things that impact our well-being – we're not taught about health and awareness in a way that relates to us.

What advice would you give to your younger self today? Or what do you wish your younger self had known, that you know today?

I'd say, in terms of hair, "Your hair is a journey." As a young person, you're trying to exist and find out who you are, and a lot of that is about outside perspective, but as you get older you get rid of that and step into your own lane and concentrate on yourself in comparison to being bothered about what your mates are doing or not doing. Wear your hair however you like and don't be afraid to try new styles. You'll find out what works for you. In terms of personal development, sit with yourself and understand who you are. Learn to develop your voice and be assured by it from a young age. "Trust yourself – you know what is best for you." As much as you might take in people's opinions or advice, take some time to think about what you want to do for yourself.

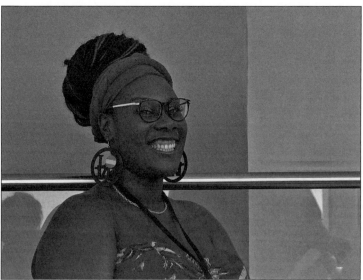

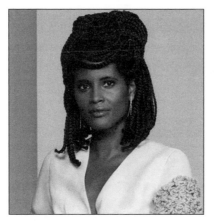

Photo: Luis Crispino

DJAMILA RIBEIRO

Brazilian human rights activist and author Djamila Ribeiro was born in the port city of Santos, Brazil. She went on to study political philosophy at Federal University of São Paulo, one of the best universities in Brazil. Djamila is now one of the most popular writers and public figures in the Afro-Brazilian women's rights movement. Her Instagram account has more than one million followers, and she regularly makes public appearances to discuss the lives of women in Brazil, a country in which people of colour experience exceptional levels of violence and prejudice. She is the author of several books, such as *Lugar de Fala* (trans: *Place of Speech*), *Quem tem medo do Feminismo Negro?* (trans: *Who's afraid of Black Feminism?*) and *Pequeno Manual Antirracista* (trans: *A Short anti-racist guide*). Her most recent book is *Cartas para minha avó* (trans: *Letters For My Grandmother*). She is also a guest professor in the journalism department at the Pontifical Catholic University of São Paulo (PUC-SP). A columnist for *Folha de S. Paulo* newspaper and *Elle* magazine, Djamila became the deputy assistant of human rights for the city of São Paulo in 2016. She was awarded the 2019 Prince Claus Award, granted by the Kingdom of the Netherlands and considered by the BBC one of the 100 most influential women in the world, the same year. In 2020, she won the Jabuti Award, the most important literature prize in Brazil. In 2021, she became the first Black Brazilian person to win the BET Awards, granted by the Black community of United States of America.

What was your go-to hairstyle as a child, and who used to do your hair?

My mother braided my hair when I was a child. But after a while, she started to straighten it when we had an event, with a hot iron, one of those that you heated up on the stove. Often it was a painful process, as it burned my scalp. On a daily basis she braided my hair, and sometimes she took me to make Kanekalon braids with hair braiders. I suffered a lot of racist abuse at school because of my hair, and for that reason I begged to use chemicals or get my hair flat ironed in the salon. My father, a member of the Black Rights Movement, would not let me, until after much insistence, he relented. And, from time to time, we straightened our hair in the salon. My grandmother lived in another city, but when I spent my vacations with her, she always braided my hair with great care.

Who was your hair inspiration growing up? Did you struggle to find Black hair inspiration?

As there were no references on TV or in magazines, coupled with the bullying I suffered at school, I wanted to straighten my hair. I didn't like to wear my hair in a natural way. Several times I put long towels on my head to simulate straight hair. The biggest children's reference on television in my childhood was a blonde woman with blue eyes who had blonde girls as assistants; it was as if Black girls did not exist. So it was a hard period, of non-acceptance, of suffering, with the imposition of such an alien beauty standard.

Who are the Black female role models in society, and how do they differ from the role models you had growing up?

In Brazil, as a consequence of the colonization process, several stereotypes were created in relation to Black women, but two are worthy of our attention: the place of subordination, reinforced in the role of the maid and that of sexualization, whose main symbol is the mulatto woman. Lelia González, an important Brazilian Black feminist, in her work "Racism and Sexism in Brazilian Society" thinks of Brazil from the point of view of these two concepts imposed on Black women.

As I said, my father was a member of the Black Rights Movement, which was very important in raising my awareness of the racial issues in society, but I lacked Black female references growing up in a place which was, often, very male-dominated. It was my mother, through Candomblé, who allowed me to have access to other representations. And then, in my late teens, when I worked for an organization called Casa da Cultura da Mulher Negra, that I met Black activists, writers and thinkers. It was a turning point in my life to be able to think about the world from those other viewpoints. And to learn to value the heritage that I came from, of maids, forcibly brought to this place because of exploitation, human oppression; women with histories, life, and who always knew the value of education.

When you were young, what beauty standards did you associate with being beautiful, and how do they differ today?

When I was young, I thought that having straight hair and fair skin was beauty. When I was very young, before going to school, I felt beautiful. My parents always reinforced how beautiful I and my brothers were. We were raised in a home where we felt good about being who we were. Everything changed when I went to school and had my first contact with institutional racism. There I was ugly, the boys didn't want to be with me at parties; I didn't have the knowledge to contest either what they said or the views of my teachers. Television confirmed what they said and, as much as my parents kept on saying how beautiful I was, it was an unfair war, and I started to dislike myself. From the Casa da Cultura da Mulher Negra (House of Culture of the Black Woman) everything changed. Ever since I got pregnant with my daughter, now 16, I have never straightened my hair again. I was able to feel the texture of my natural hair again after the age of 25. But I think that this building of self-esteem goes beyond the aesthetic issue, which is important, without a doubt, but it has to do directly with having access to Black feminist books and media, and the expansion of my worldview from them. And also with my return to Candomblé as an adult. My daughter has never straightened her hair,

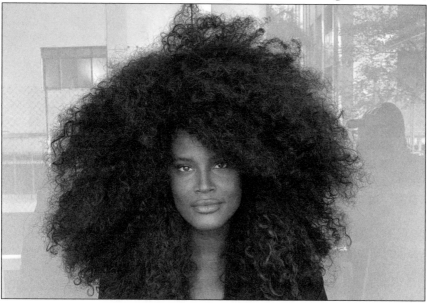

Photo: Ale de Souza

she didn't have many of the issues I had, so I see it as a process of healing and deliverance.

At what age were you made to feel like your hair was different? Tell us about that experience, what it felt like and how you navigated that?

At around six years old, when I went to school. It was a very tough process, of suffering a lot of abuse at school and being the butt of jokes and acquiring a quasi-obsession with straightening my hair.

What age were you when you started to make your own hair decisions, what were those decisions, and why did you choose the style you did?

At 24, when I got pregnant with my daughter. It is important to note that I did not stop straightening because of an awareness process, but because I had become pregnant and could not use chemicals during this period. I usually say that my daughter helped me in this process, since from there I started having a healthy relationship with my hair. I started to braid again and did the big chop. I found its texture again. Today I use braids, in a natural way, but for me there is the political issue of not straightening. I do not judge women who straighten their hair. I don't think there is one standard that should be imposed on women, and we also cannot put others down. That's why I am careful to look at other Black women with compassion. But I haven't straightened my own hair in 16 years. I like to see myself with the aesthetics of Black beauty which I was denied for a long time. And I love the versatility that curly hair offers; I'm able to create a series of hairstyles and discover myself in this process with my hairdresser.

Do you have any experiences where your hair had a major effect on something in your life?

Not wanting to leave the house in my teens due to not feeling my hair was beautiful, not letting people in my inner circle touch my hair. It was a long process until I felt comfortable with it.

What part does your hair play in your life today? What in your "hair story" helped shape that?

A very important role as it concerns my identity and the construction of my identity. It is not merely aesthetic. It is a statement, however, at the same time, in my intimate moments it is not something that worries me – not having an impeccable hairstyle. I am not a doll, I am a human being. If the root is showing in the braids, I don't bother anymore. It's just my hair growing and it's OK.

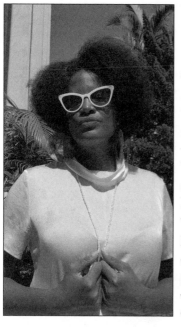

What do you think about how brands situate themselves in the narrative of black hair? What more do you think could be done?

The concept of the "perfect curl", for example seems outdated. My hair is curly, but I found it very difficult to find products for my hair, even those brands that said they were designed for our hair. It is necessary to break away from the idea of homogenization and respect plurality. We need to see more Black women with dark skin in advertising, with different types of hair. To go beyond a pseudo inclusive discourse.

What do you think of the differences between the way Black men and Black women are treated in society when it comes to standards of beauty?

There are many differences, despite the similarities. Racism is structural, it structures all social relations and has a preponderant role in the construction of the beautiful, of what society perceives as beautiful. And it affects as many men as women. However, when it is intertwined with sexism, then we begin to see the importance of the intersectional approach. There is a greater pressure to conform for Black women with regard to their hair and body. While all women suffer to adapt to what society has stipulated as the "perfect body", Black women also have to deal with the racist and sexist stereotype in Brazil about the "mulatto", the light Black woman, with curves, who is sexualized. And there is also the archetype of the "Black mother", the fat and asexual Black woman, who takes care of everyone. As much as Black men are also sexualized, these reductive concepts of women affect Black women more negatively, or as the Brazilian Black intellectual, Luiza Bairros said, "we carry the brand".

What more do you think needs to be done to empower Black women, particulary regarding hair and beauty?

I think it is necessary to work on these issues at school. As much as we have a law in Brazil, created in 2003, which changed the Law of Guidelines and Bases of Education to include African and Afro-Brazilian history in schools, it is not implemented as it should be. It is necessary that Black girls have positive references to help build their identities and self-esteem. That we must demand that media and entertainment in general show more diverse images. I always insist on this project of raising awareness.

What advice would you give to your younger self today? Or, what do you wish your younger self had known, that you know today?

I would tell young Djamila not to believe the racism discourse, lest she suffer so much and waste so much time thinking about it. But I think I have healed young Djamila by saying all this to my daughter Thulane. Young Djamila was healed when she saw her daughter feel as beautiful as she is. My awareness and discovery process was passed on.

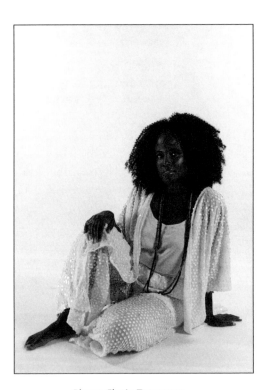

Photo: Flavio Teperman

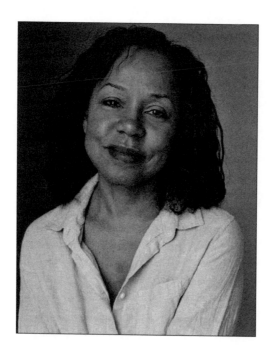

VIVIENNE ROCHESTER

Vivienne Rochester is of Caribbean and British Heritage, and if you go back to another generation, there is some Indian ancestry too. She is an actor with many years of experience working at The Royal Shakespeare Company, The Royal Court, The Salisbury Playhouse, The Apollo Theatre, The Menier Chocolate Factory and many other theatres. Her TV work includes *Casualty*, *The Bill* and a 20-minute monologue *Window of Vulnerability* for The BBC.

She has worked as Head of Drama, Dance and Speech for City Lit from 2001–2015 and as a Speech and Drama examiner and Drama School Assessor at Trinity College. She is also a trained psychotherapist.

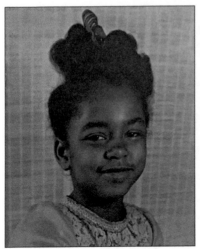

What was your go-to hairstyle as a child, and who used to do your hair?

My mother did my hair – I wasn't allowed to. Whenever there was anything special on, she would twist it into ringlets – otherwise, I think she just plaited it and put it up. When I began to look after it, I would have it in bunches or pulled back, or it would be set in rollers when I wanted to achieve a special hairstyle. My mother didn't allow me to straighten my hair for quite a long time, that was a no-no, so I started doing it in secret when I was a late teenager. By the end of my teens, I could straighten my hair, but it was definitely taboo for a long time. I think my hair was slightly frizzier than it is now. I remember going to school one day, and I had it parted on the side, and I remember my junior schoolteacher telling me it looked like a Russian hat.

You stopped relaxing your hair a couple of years ago. What made you stop?

Probably several reasons. It was a conscious thing – I was destroying my hair. But also, I thought it was just time that I stopped. When I was a kid, I used to put a towel over my head and pretend that my hair swung. As time went on, I tried a curly perm. So I've gone through the fashions and the fads, but now I'm with the movement that we should be more ourselves. As I am an actor, it's quite difficult. For instance, I came in as a guest to play a customs officer about 10 years ago. I went into the audition, and my hair was straight – I used to have my hair in a bob, and I got the audition. I've always tended to relax my hair, but I'd let it be natural in the holidays – just to give it a rest. So when I came in for the costume fitting because it was the summer, it wasn't straight, and the director was horrified. He said, "I can't have your hair like that. I don't know what's happened." Then he tried to explain to me about how I had my hair before. He said, "I want to see your hair straight, with a fringe". I just thought, isn't that interesting? I think that certain roles certainly expect your hair to look closely like the hair of a Caucasian. As I tend to play professional roles, I think that's what the association is – that hair should be sleek. It pissed me off, but I just got my straighteners out and did it. It did make me cross that suddenly I was not the same person, with the same worth. This is why our hair is such a big thing – because a white person can do whatever, but the association is, the more we look like them, the more acceptable we are. And the more we are like ourselves, the more 'other' we are.

Who was your hair inspiration growing up? Did you struggle to find Black hair inspiration?

Diana Ross, Tina Turner and people like that were fabulous, and they were quintessentially Black. But I'll tell you who I liked, and I wrote to her to tell her and asked her what products she used – Cleo Laine. I loved her hair, I thought, I want my hair to look like that. When I was much younger, it was Cathy McGowan from *Ready Steady Go*; long straight hair with a fringe. Of course, when I began to really look at things, I began to look at people like Angela Davis and the Civil Rights people. And *Hair* the musical – with all of the big hair. I did have an Afro at one point – small, but it was there. I was in New York for a bit, and it was like, "Woah!" I'd only ever been surrounded by white people in the UK, really – at school and at college and university – and when I went to the States as a contemporary ballet dancer I was surrounded by Black people. I was very odd in my family – the people in my family are all maths and history-based – and I was the 'arts' one. When I got to New York – I remember it to this day, it is a really formative memory – I was at a party completely surrounded by artists, and they were all Black, all shades, from different countries. We were all sitting around – somebody had a guitar, somebody was speaking poetry – and we had this wonderful huge bowl of African food we were eating from with our hands. And I just remember having this physical, cellular, deep feeling that I was in this huge embrace because here were people that looked like me and were like me. It felt like home because, until that moment, I had not ever recognized myself in others. I'm tearing up a little bit – it was, and still is, a really significant, important memory. It's to do with being who I am and having that endorsement that I'm not odd – that I have a tribe.

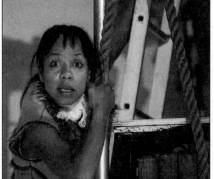

At what age were you made to feel like your hair was different? Tell us about that experience, what it felt like and how you navigated that?

I remember in school kids asking me about why the palms of my hands were white. I don't particularly remember anything about hair, but I knew my hair was problematic. Now, I've embraced the hassle. I do what my mother used to do – I twist it and then untwist it. There was a time when I twisted it and just kept it twisted, and it was curly, which I quite liked. But then my hair started to break. If I just went to bed and didn't comb it – it would tangle. Now, I have to contend with it going grey.

Who are the Black female role models in society, and how do they differ from the role models you had growing up?

They are more visible now: Michelle Obama, Oprah Winfrey, Beyoncé, Toni Morrison, Maya Angelou, Chimamanda Ngozi Adiche. The people I have huge respect for are people who have intelligence and integrity. Right now, the quality of our leadership is really poor. I think of Trump, Boris... The pandemic proves that there aren't any barriers. Let's get over ourselves – there aren't any borders, so why are we going through Brexit? This country has a ridiculous idea of itself based on its legacy, history and colonizations of continents, so it hangs on to that. Still, it's a tiny little country and island, and there is no place for an isolated island of power and influence, greed and pillage any longer. White men still run it, and they still employ who they look like, who they see. So that is prevalent, and it's very difficult to change that. All we can keep doing is smashing through the glass ceiling to create change. If you turn on your TV and look at the adverts, suddenly there's an awful lot of Black people and mixed relationships in the adverts, so there is a concerted effort – in particular, because of the Black Lives Matter movement. It woke up quite a lot of industries; I'm hoping that it's not just lip service – there's already kickback from it. I just hope that change is actually going to be built on. The same thing goes on and on and on, and the attitudes remain. They go in for meaningless token gestures, jump on the ethical bandwagon for two seconds, but nothing changes. So that's the fight. But the good thing is that Black people are working through it. For instance, a Chaplain to the Queen is a Black woman [Rose Hudson-Wilkin]. So we are striving and getting there, I just think society, in general, is always surprised when somebody stands up, and then you get backlash. Like with the Sainsbury's [Christmas] advert with the Black family – there's a section of the population that doesn't want it, but they don't understand that a large part of this country was built on slave labour. I think it's human nature to be frightened of the "other"; you project your fears onto them. They don't acknowledge our presence through history, and we have been here a very, very long time. But they don't document it. And half of the people running around here have Black blood in their veins; they just don't know it!

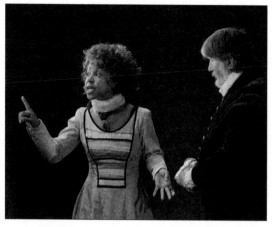

When you were young, what beauty standards did you associate with being beautiful, and how do they differ today?

I think about all the white people with their big lips and big bums – they're copying Black lips and Black bums – and they acknowledge that we are the models of that now, so I think it's changed dramatically. The likes of Viola Davis – I've been watching her avidly in *How to Get Away With Murder*, she's gone through every look in that show – natural, beaten up – everything. It's an extraordinary thing. She'll go to bed with the bonnet on her head. She shows every aspect, every look that we have, and she has been brave enough to show it – rather than just the glamorous weaves. I like that; the strength of mind and purpose to expose all of the different sides to ourselves. That's the thing about us, and I quote Oprah Winfrey: "I come as one, but I stand as ten thousand." There is such a diverse range within ourselves, and what's good is that there's more exposure to that. The idea of beauty, I still think it's largely white and petite, but it's changing. I think the fact that someone like Winnie Harlow can be so successful is great. It is less rigid than it was.

Do you have any experiences where your hair had a major effect on something in your life?

Not really, but that's because I conformed. I straightened my hair. I did what they wanted me to do. I dressed like my hair – appropriately. I'd do what was easy. I was aware that I shouldn't really be doing it, not least because of the potential damage. Hence I would have those summer holiday breaks where my hair would be natural. But I'm not doing my hair like that anymore.

What do you think about how brands situate themselves in the narrative of Black hair? What more do you think could be done?

Because we consider ourselves to have problematic hair, they have exploited that. The brands have very much been responsible for how we see ourselves and our hair. I just think people will exploit each other, and it's just the age we live in – an age of complete self-interest.

What do you think of the differences between the way Black men and Black women are treated in society when it comes to standards of beauty?

In terms of beauty, the net is much wider for a man than for a woman. The lighter the skin colour for women, the more accepted you are – that isn't quite the case for Black men. And you'll see Black men and white women being promoted – you don't see that so much the other way around. But it is beginning to change.

What more do you think needs to be done to empower Black women, particularly regarding hair and beauty?

Give them a voice, see them and recognize them. Black women have so much to offer, such a history of survival, courage, fortitude and perseverance. They are a huge resource of wealth and are very capable. I don't care what walk of life they come from; if you want something done, ask a Black woman.

What advice would you give to your younger self today? Or what do you wish your younger self had known, that you know today?

I'd tell her that we are gorgeous and talented and intelligent, and as good as everybody else.

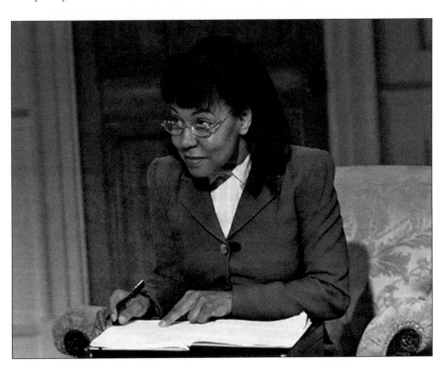

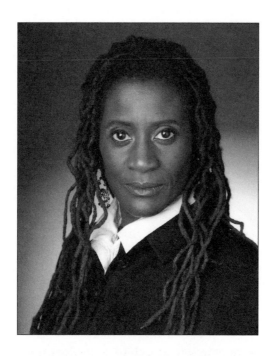

KADIJA GEORGE SESAY

Kadija George Sesay Hon. FRSL, FRSA is a Sierra Leonean British literary activist, short story writer and poet, and the publisher and managing editor of the magazine *SABLE LitMag*. Her work has earned her many awards and nominations, including the Cosmopolitan Woman of Achievement in 1994, Candace Woman of Achievement in 1996, The Voice Community Award in Literature in 1999 and the Millennium Woman of the Year in 2000.

She graduated with a degree in West African Studies from Birmingham University, then worked as a Black Literature Development co-ordinator for Centreprise in the 90s, where she launched and ran the newspaper *Calabash*. In 2001–2015 she founded and published *SABLE LitMag*. Sesay has also edited and co-edited several books, including *Burning Words, Flaming Images: Poems and Short Stories by Writers of African Descent* (1996), *IC3: The Penguin Book of New Black Writing in Britain* (with Courttia Newland, 2000), *Dance the Guns to Silence: 100 Poems for Ken Saro-Wiwa* (Flipped Eye Publishing, 2005), and (as Kadija George) *Six Plays by Black and Asian Women Writers* (Aurora Metro Books, 1993), *Write Black, Write British: From Post Colonial to Black*

British Literature (Hansib Publications, 2005). She is the co-author of *This is the Canon: Decolonise Your Bookshelf in 50 Books*, (Quercus Publishing, 2021).

In 2007 she created the first SABLE Literary Festival in The Gambia, where she now programmes the Mboka Festival of Arts, Culture & Sport which she co- founded in 2016. She is Publications Manager of Peepal Tree Press's writer development programme, Inscribe, alongside fellow poet Dorothea Smartt.

Sesay's first full collection of poems, entitled *Irki,* was published in 2013. Her poetry, short stories and essays have appeared in a range of publications, including the 2019 anthology *New Daughters of Africa,* edited by Margaret Busby.

Sesay is a doctoral researcher in Black British Publishing and Pan-Africanism. She was appointed Member of the Order of the British Empire (MBE) in the 2020 Birthday Honours for services to Publishing and awarded an Honorary Fellowship of the Royal Society of Literature in 2021 for services to Literature.

What was your go-to hairstyle as a child, and who used to do your hair?

My hair was threaded with black cotton to lay flat on my scalp for school, to keep hair as neat as possible. Very traditional in West Africa. Now there are many more innovative, creative versions of threading. I went back to Sierra Leone for the first time when I was 12 years old, and they had plastic thread used with black wool extensions. I loved it and never wanted to take it out, but there wasn't anyone my mother knew who could do it for me when we got back to the UK. Until a few years ago, girls in government schools in Ghana had to keep their hair cropped short. There are pros and cons to this, which is a major discussion in itself.

My mum used to do my hair. She would visit us every two weeks (we were privately fostered as children) so she would do it at the weekend when I would rather be out playing with friends!

When we went out for family occasions like weddings and christenings, my hair was hot combed. The memories of that are Vaseline, that was put on the combs. (You usually needed to have at least two different sizes of combs). You'd have burn marks around the edges of your scalp, on the back of the neck, the tops of your ears… but it made your hair temporarily straight (as long as you didn't sweat too much or get rained on) and it could be styled

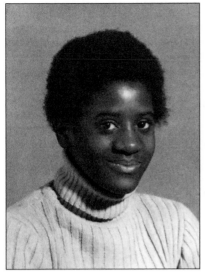

in various ways. I remember having a parting on one side! Just the fact that I could feel my hair without my fingers getting caught up in curls was some kind of magic.

Who was your hair inspiration growing up? Did you struggle to find Black hair inspiration?

Hair was often the cause of anxiety and depression. My hair never seemed to grow that long, so it was difficult to style it in any fashion, and that was part of being seen as attractive.

Who are the Black female role models in society, and how do they differ from the role models you had growing up?

There were less Black female role models than there are now when I was growing up, and only famous people were seen as role models rather than women working in business or the community for example. Today there are Black role models in different areas of life and work. I know a lot of women I would call role models, such as my sister, who are simply formidable women. A role model for me, for several years, although she is less public now, is Susan L. Taylor who was the editor for *Essence* magazine for almost 20 years, before running the Essence Music Festival. Sonia Sanchez, Margaret Busby, Oprah Winfrey. There are women who have recently passed who I have a lot of admiration for: Cicely Tyson, Winnie Madikizela-Mandela, Nawal el Saadawi, Buchi Emecheta and Jessica Huntley. They are all role models for different things they have said or done. I 'll leave it there. My list could fill a page.

When you were young, what beauty standards did you associate with being beautiful, and how do they differ today?

Dark-skinned (as all the women in my family are). Natural hair, as only older women wore wigs when I was younger, so in my mind I associated wigs with getting old. Young women didn't wear wigs so natural hair was the only option I knew – managing it was the challenge. At the time when perming or conditioning hair was seen as part of the beauty package, it was associated with a lot of angst, and I couldn't seem to justify in my mind having that much angst to 'look beautiful' by other people's standards.

People tried to force other beauty standards on me in subtle ways, but I was too naïve to understand what that was all about, so in the end, I just ignored it.

At what age were you made to feel like your hair was different? Tell us about that experience, what it felt like and how you navigated that?

I realized that my hair was a fascination when I was at infants' school as I was the only Black girl in the school (and my brother was the only Black boy). A boy in arts and craft class cut my hair. I didn't say anything, and I didn't actually realize what had happened until my mum came to do my hair at the weekend; she started to thread it and my hair came out in her hands in a clump. She was so upset. When I told her what had happened, my parents demanded to speak to the boy's parents, which was quite amusing as his father was a vicar. I had a thinned patch at the back of my head for at least 20 years after that. That was the real disaster. I wrote a poem about the incident.

What age were you when you started to make your own hair decisions? What were those decisions, and why did you choose the style you did?

Probably in the first year of secondary school. I can't remember at what age I started to make my own hair decisions. I think it was more like a combination of my mother being too busy working and saying I need to take responsibility to do my own hair and no longer having my hair threaded. What I do remember, is that, too often I tried to style a mini Afro – and it was mini as my hair didn't grow that long, and I spent many tearful mornings trying to get both sides even.

It was probably in my second or third year of secondary school (when I was 12 or 13) that my Aunt Isatu arrived from Sierra Leone and lived nearby. She is brilliant at braiding lots of lovely hairstyles. I loved them. I remember that she did my hair for a few years and that is when it started to slowly grow longer.

What part does your hair play in your life today? What in your "hair story" helped shape that?

I'm a very lazy hair person – which is why I have locs, but to keep locs in good condition, it still takes work. For many years in my twenties and thirties my hair was low to my scalp and then I started to dye it golden bronze all over or in patches. I loved it. I didn't realize though that with that hairstyle, people thought I was a lesbian – I had no idea. Probably the reason why I didn't have boyfriends which I didn't realize until several years later.

So for years I had my hair skinned as I really couldn't be bothered to do anything with my hair as the stress and anxiety that it caused me when growing up was still fresh, but short hair was the same thing – to keep it neat and tidy, you have to get it done regularly and I went from hairdressers to barbers – barbers were less judgmental. If I went to a hairdresser, they always tried to make me have my hair conditioned and permed. I felt so intimidated. I had my hair cooked for about two to three years in my life and hated it about eighty per cent of the time. I saw it as just a more expensive, chemicalized version of hot combing that remained straight for a longer period of time. Then I started to have it braided with extensions. That was life-changing for me. I felt that I could finally embrace and enjoy 'hair'. It was done really well at a house of a friend. She was great. I kept my hair braided with extensions for a very long time until I decided to locks it.

What do you think about how brands situate themselves in the narrative of Black hair? What more do you think could be done?

The problem is that none of the big name brands that make money out of Black women's hair are Black-owned. That may have changed since the time I was involved with things like the Black Hair and Beauty Show – but then, I was only really involved to approach companies for advertising for the Black magazines I worked with. Wherever I can get natural organic oils for my hair, that is what I use. I used to go to Back To Eden in South London – Cynthia was the first loctician in London and she also used to have natural hair products rather than stuff for chemicalized hair. There are so many more natural hair salons available now and that is not seen as unusual – that's a good thing! When I was younger if you wore your hair naturally you were seen as unsophisticated and "ugly". That's changed so much now, thank goodness, but not everywhere.

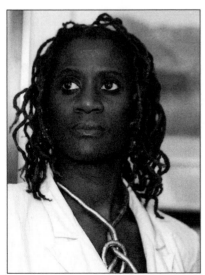

Photo: Victor Dlamini

There are still Black women – of all ages – who think that they only look beautiful with long, straight hair, whether that is natural or false hair. As children, when we went out to play, girls would fit the neck of a buttoned up cardigan on their heads, like a hat and let an arm flap down on either side. We would pretend it was our long, 'white girl' hair and swing the arms back and forth as though we were flicking our hair. Bernardine Evaristo writes about this in her book, *Lara*. It's such a strong, funny memory.

Black hair products are the most obvious examples of products that millions of Black pounds are spent on,

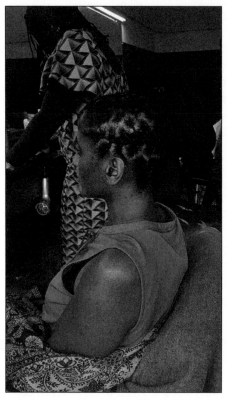

with the Black community receiving little, if any, of the profits. It's quite depressing and so I try not to think about it too much.

Most of the time, I now get my hair done when I am abroad, and ask around for the best loctitian available, and then I will always go to the same one. The reminders of intimidation at hairdressing salons have remained with me. I get it done mainly when I am in Africa. It's much better value and the service and outcome is excellent. When I am in The Gambia, Sadjo my hairstylist gives me a wash, scalp massage, retwist and style – for the price of a sandwich!

I've really missed not getting my hair done properly during the pandemic and I'm rubbish at doing it myself.

What more do you think needs to be done to empower Black women, particulary regarding hair and beauty?

Ownership. Black hair is big business, but how much of it do we own? I'm not really into human hair wigs and extensions of whatever colour. I think they are fine for fun but not for permanent use – I don't get it. The history of Black women's hair though has its own trajectory of colonial (mis) use and (mis) understanding. Maybe I need to start a 'Decolonize your hair' campaign!

What advice would you give to your younger self today? Or, what do you wish your younger self had known, that you know today?

I wish I had locksed my hair earlier in my life. Dreadlocks are how our hair naturally grows but locksing is a political statement, too, and even though I was politically aware, I didn't really understand the depths of it and the links to dreadlocks and our African heritage. So now I keep my hair locksed because of the politics around the issues of African people and our hair as much as with the practicality of it.

Anything else you'd like to add?

I didn't expect and always said I wouldn't write poems about hair because I feel that the focus on hair is too much of a distraction away from more important things in life that we need to deal with. I've joked before when I've read my hair poems in public that Black women could have a conference on hair – it is never just a five minute conversation.

Ideally, if I'd been brave, I would have been bald. I'm just too busy to spend precious time dealing with my hair these days and also it's because it's been distressing during the formative years of my life, and because those who made me feel worse about my hair were other Black women. I was made to feel that I was not a woman or not attractive if I didn't spend money on my hair… so I went in the opposite direction and decided not to care about it at all. I often wear head wraps. Fashion aside, I think everyone should wear their hair naturally, in dreadlocks, braids, as an Afro or free flow. Or go bald.

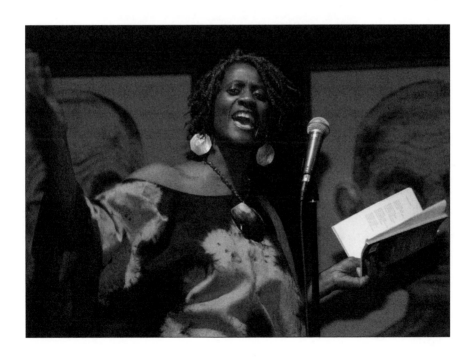

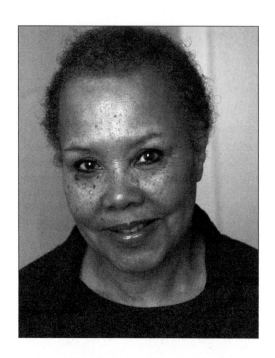

CLEO SYLVESTRE

Cleo Sylvestre is an English actress in film, stage and television. She was the first Black woman ever to play a leading role at the National Theatre in London.

She was brought up in Euston, North London, and educated at Camden School for Girls, briefly attending the Italia Conti Academy of Theatre Arts, and while training as a Primary School Teacher, left to pursue acting. Her West End debut was at Wyndham's Theatre in *Wise Child* (1967) by Simon Gray, in which she starred alongside Sir Alec Guinness and was nominated most promising new actress. She was the first Black actress in a leading role at the National Theatre in *The National Health* (1969) by Peter Nichols followed by seasons at The Young Vic including tours to Broadway and Mexico. She has performed in a wide range of theatre productions including touring with Northern Broadsides and Oxford Playhouse. For 20 years until June 2016, Cleo was joint Artistic Director of the award-winning Rosemary Branch Theatre.

Film/TV: Cleo was in Ken Loach's films *Cathy Come Home, Up The Junction* and *Poor Cow* and has acted in numerous TV shows from *Grange Hill*, to presenting *Playschool*, and guesting in the Christmas 2020 special of *All Creatures Great and Small*. She made several shorts for Isaac Julien including *Vagabondia* (Turner Prize shortlist), was in *Kidulthood* and *Tube Tales* (dir. Jude Law) and *Paddington*. In 2019 Cleo received the Screen Nation Trailblazer Award.

Music: Having made a record with the (then unknown) Rolling Stones while at school, she recently returned to her first love, music, forming the blues band, Honey B Mama & Friends, who have appeared at the Queen Elizabeth Hall and the Ealing Blues Festival among many other venues.

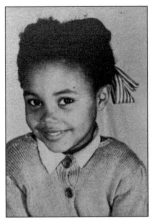

What was your go-to hairstyle as a child, and who used to do your hair?

As a child my hair was usually in two plaits made by my mother who was born and brought up in Yorkshire and of mixed heritage. I used to dread it when my surrogate father (who was from Trinidad) did my hair. It looked amazing after, but he was not as gentle as my mum so it would hurt while he was doing it. I remember sitting on the floor and him telling me not to wriggle and me trying not to cry with the pain.

Who was your hair inspiration growing up? Did you struggle to find Black hair inspiration?

My hair inspiration growing up was from white film stars of the 40s and 50s, usually American. Black representation in the media was virtually non-existent. Television was not present in many households – in fact I was about 15 years old before we had a TV, so I would go to the cinema where the actors were mostly exclusively white. Also, it was rare to see people in magazines and newspapers at that time who were not white.

Who are the Black female role models in society, and how do they differ from the role models you had growing up?

This is a difficult question as there are now so many younger Black female role models. However, the ones I've chosen are those who are older and have succeeded without probably having role models of their own. For example, Margaret Busby, the publisher who edited the seminal *Daughters of Africa,* Chi-chi Nwanoku founder of the Chineke! Orchestra, Jackie Kay the poet, Joan Armatrading and Dame Elizabeth Anionwu. I wasn't aware of any Black female role models when I was growing up.

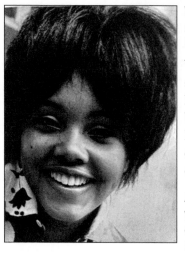

When you were young, what beauty standards did you associate with being beautiful, and how do they differ today?

When I was young, to be beautiful was associated with being white-skinned and having European (i.e. not frizzy or Afro) hair because this is what was portrayed in adverts. Fortunately, today there has been a sea change and it is accepted that all ethnicities can be beautiful.

At what age were you made to feel like your hair was different? Tell us about that experience, what it felt like and how you navigated that?

When I went to school at five, I realized my hair was different, prior to that I hadn't really thought about it. A boy on my first day at school called me "Blackie", and I realized I was a different colour from all the other children. My reaction was to go to my mother's rag bag (most people then saved odd bits of material for patching etc). I then tied bits of material to my hair so I could feel what it was like for my hair to move about and toss over my shoulders.

What age were you when you started to make your own hair decisions, what were those decisions, and why did you choose the style you did?

I started to make my own hair decisions around 15 when I was at school and had a Saturday job, so I could afford to go to a hairdressers. I had my hair straightened first of all with a heated comb, but if it rained, that was trouble, and it reverted to being frizzy. I then had it straightened with chemicals which were excruciatingly painful. I wanted to have long straight hair with a fringe so I could be like all my friends. Later, I chose a Mary Quant bob.

Do you have any experiences where your hair had a major effect on something in your life?

Not long after starting school in 1950, I was playing in the street near Euston, with my (white) friend who lived next door. There were not many cars around in those days and we were delighted when a big chauffeur-driven car pulled up. The driver got out and opened the door for the smartly dressed woman in the back. She rushed towards me and ran her fingers through my hair asking her companion to get out and do the same. This reinforced what I was told my first day at school, that I was different from most people I knew, apart from my mother and father.

What part does your hair play in your life today? What in your "hair story" helped shaped that?

Today, I am the happiest I have ever been with my hair. It's natural, no straightening, weaves, extensions or dyeing. Such a feeling of freedom. I was always uncomfortable from an ethical viewpoint, having extensions and hearing stories about how people in the Far East would sell their hair to raise money. Regarding straighteners, I decided enough was enough having nasty chemicals on my scalp and the pain associated with it.

What do you think about how brands situate themselves in the narrative of Black hair? What more do you think could be done?

Things have improved, but there still seems to be a tendency for brands to get Black people to feel that only European hair is desirable and to push having extensions, weaves etc. When I look at the ingredients of some products, I feel that some brands should be more environmentally friendly.

What do you think of the differences between the way Black men and Black women are treated in society when it comes to standards of beauty?

I feel men are allowed to be far more natural, whereas there is still a pressure for women to aspire to European type hair and lighter skin. However, there have been recent changes and, thankfully, it is now far more acceptable for Black men and women to be proud of how they naturally look and not trying to conceal or alter their innate beauty.

What more do you think needs to be done to empower Black women, particularly regarding hair and beauty?

Advertising needs to be more responsible and celebrate Blackness, not trying to get their customers to hide or disguise it. Reports of schoolchildren being excluded for wearing Afros, braids, locs etc. needs to be addressed.

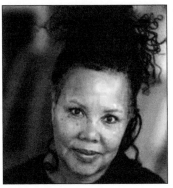

What advice would you give to your younger self today? Or, what do you wish your younger self had known, that you know today?

Be yourself and listen to your inner voice. I wish my younger self had known that there were millions of girls like me all over the world and I was not alone.

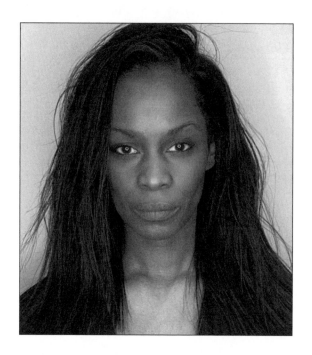

CARRYL THOMAS

Carryl is an English actress who grew up in South London and studied Musical Theatre at Mountview Academy of Theatre Arts.

Carryl has just completed filming for the new series of *Silent Witness* for the BBC and is currently playing Cara Robinson in ITV's *Emmerdale*. She began her career in West End musicals performing in award-winning shows such as *My Fair Lady* and *Our House,* and created the role of Keisha in the world premiere of *Flashdance,* directed by Tony award-winning director Kenny Leon and choreographed by Arlene Phillips.

Channel 5's soap, *Family Affairs,* provided her with the opportunity to take on the role of troubled teen, Kelly Boulter, for which she received British Soap And Screen Nation Award nominations. Carryl subsequently joined the cast of *The Sarah Jane Adventures* for Doctor Who Productions, and made guest appearances in *Holby City.* Other work includes filming a new crime series from the producers of *CSI* and *Law and Order* starring Jean Reno in Paris, commercials, Royal Variety performances and voiceovers.

As a busy mother of four boys, Carryl combines working as an actress, with teaching Dance, Speech and Drama, and runs her own part-time school and agency for children.

What was your go-to hairstyle as a child, and who used to do your hair?

In primary school it was always plaited, so I'd have cornrow plaits or loose plaits. It was a Sunday evening ritual where my mum would have my hair washed and conditioned, and my aunts and my cousins would all come round, have tea together, watch *The Cosby Show*, and all the girls would then get their hair braided for the week for school. For secondary school my mum started giving me the freedom to do what I wanted with my hair, and I literally just scraped it up into a ponytail thinking it was cool, but obviously it wasn't cool at all! So I embraced it but still tried to tame it. Back then I went to a private girls' school in Wimbledon and there weren't many Black girls, so, to wear your own hair as it was intended, I would take a guess and say it wouldn't have necessarily been tolerated. Even these days girls wear Afros or certain hairstyles at school and get told to go back, so looking back to when I was at school 20 to 30 years ago, I'm almost certain it would have been the same response.

When you look back on that now, do you regret not trying to embrace your natural hair in that environment?

One hundred per cent, because I think whatever we do as young people sets the tone for us as adults. Whether it's us trying to hide it or someone else trying to stifle it, it's damaging. I think it's left me a bit safe with my experimentation and with my pride. I look at my children and they've got the most amazing Afros, and I kind of feel myself wanting to show off their manes and make it a thing, but unfortunately it wasn't there for me.

Who was your hair inspiration growing up? Did you struggle to find Black hair inspiration?

I have loads of aunties and cousins, and they've all got wonderful hair and do a lot with it, but in terms of media there was nothing I can recall, except for *The Cosby Show*, *The Fresh Prince of Belair* and *A Different World*. I would buy magazines – there was no Googling back then – and look at all of the hairstyles. We had *Ebony* and *Black Hair*, and I would literally cut out pics to keep in my diary so I could secretly try new things in my bedroom at the weekend. You tried it and you felt great, but you didn't wear it out, you just kept it to yourself. Not because anyone said you couldn't, but it wasn't visible so it kind of set the tone that it was meant to be a secret. I feel crazy saying that out loud now, but that's exactly how it felt back then. It was the same with make-up. They say it's supply and demand for a demographic, but surely you have to supply it first to know there's no demand?

Who are the Black female role models in society, and how do they differ from the role models you had growing up?

The ones growing up were my aunties, my sister, my cousins – the women in my life. I don't recall there being many Black British role models on the scene. But now I turn to artists in the entertainment industry. We've also got Kamala Harris – she's definitely a huge role model in all walks of life. There are actresses like Thandie Newton – who's British and very much embraces Black culture and hair – and she's proud of her heritage. Angela Bassett is a great actress who I love, and I love Beyoncé – she's my hero. It's important to see yourself in a role model from all aspects. My family are made up of women from diverse backgrounds and it's important we stand together not just as women, but as women of colour.

When you were young, what beauty standards did you associate with being beautiful, and how do they differ today?

It was all about if you didn't have long hair, light skin or light eyes, you weren't looked at. If you weren't thin, tall. It didn't matter what you had between your ears, your brain and the power of knowledge, it was all about the aesthetic, and aesthetics that weren't very healthy, balanced or based on reality. Naomi Campbell was the one supermodel we all knew growing up and she was great, and yes, she's very beautiful, but you shouldn't have to be beautiful to be acknowledged, or to be heard and given a voice.

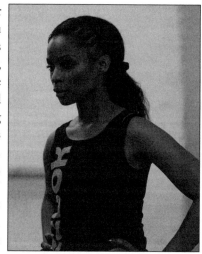

A lot of our shape is down to our genetics. I was told in ballet class: "You won't ever make it because your bottom's too big". But then you look at Alvin Ailey, and all the Alvin Ailey dancers – they've all got big, strong bottoms and they're all fantastic dancers. So it was very damaging growing up for me because there was nothing in my time that encouraged you. And our parents came over from various countries, so I think there was a lot of fear with them to speak up. My mum was very quiet – she wanted the best for us. We grew up in South London, in not the best area, and she worked three jobs to make sure all three of us went to private schools. Then she had to fight at school to make sure we were heard and that we weren't overlooked – because my brother and sister were very bright she used to have to fight to make sure that it was noted. It wasn't enough that they got into the school, she had to fight all the way through to get them to university. We think it's hard now, but it was much harder back then. They brought their children into this society and felt compelled to fit in, but nowadays I tell my children, "You don't have to fit in, you just have to be a good person and do what's right." There are many more role models now because there's more freedom to be an individual. Opportunities are endless. I would say it's near impossible for young people today to feel as trapped as I did when I was younger.

At what age were you made to feel like your hair was different? Tell us about that experience, what it felt like and how you navigated that?

Haircare was a big thing in my house, so we had all of the oils and the greases, we plaited and washed our hair regularly, and I was given an education from day one. I remember asking to have my hair relaxed because all my cousins had their hair relaxed. When I got a bit older my mum sourced out a really good hairdresser and took me along, and the hairdresser took my hair out and said: "I'm not going to relax your hair – you have really good hair and I don't think it's the best thing for you. In my professional experience, you're a child, so just leave it." I'm really grateful for that because I feel that made me learn more and really invest my time in how to treat my hair and be versatile with it, because even to this day now, I have never relaxed it. Going to school and having swimming lessons was when I was made to feel different. A teacher once said to me when I got my cream out to do swimming, "We haven't got time to do that." This was in the 80s. Some of the girls were lucky enough to just tie their hair and leave the swimming school, but if my hair wasn't in plaits, I'd have to brush it or do something to it, because otherwise it would just get matted, but again, I wasn't allowed to do that. I think that's the reason why I can't swim – I was so hurt and scarred and embarrassed by the experience that I never went back. There would be every illness I could think of every Tuesday to not go swimming, so I never learned.

In your profession do you often get people handling your hair who really don't know what they're doing?

Yeah. In my very first job I had a lovely girl called Caroline and she knew because she asked questions and went and studied off her own back, but it wasn't readily available for training as part of the company, which is a shame because they all go and do training on various things, but it's never on Afro hair. When I went to France to do a film the French just seemed to do it; presumably it's because there's a big Black community there and also because the make-up artists were Black and mixed-raced, so they knew what they were doing. Fairly recently I had a make-up artist on *Emmerdale* who went and trained with Kamanzaa, a Black hair and beauty educator, so she knew everything – I arrived and she had all the products, and she asked me what I preferred: would I like KeraCare or something else? And I was like, "Yes! Yes, I love KeraCare," and it was just lovely that she knew. I haven't had any direct problems – my biggest problems have probably been with make-up, with getting the colour right. We had a make-up session when I was leaving drama school. As the only Black girl in my year – and the lady came with the biggest kit, but with only one shade of Black, which wasn't my shade – I had to sit there and watch while everyone else got made up. There are so many brands out there now, and there are so many tutorials, we shouldn't have to go and do our make-up ourselves – if you work for a company then you deserve to have the training. But if there isn't any training, the more people who take a stand and go out and source it for themselves means there might then be recognition to say, there's a hole here, we need to have a little training camp where we can regularly assess how to cut Black hair and curly hair, what products work on textured hair – does this person like water in their products; is it oil-based only? There should be more training and it should be standard.

What part does your hair play in your life today?

It still plays a very safe part. I think a lot of my safety in my upbringing has sort of clung on to me. But being able to take a headshot and present myself differently is my time to play and show who else I can be. If I was to wear my Afro, sadly, they don't see a blank canvas, and that really infuriates me, because

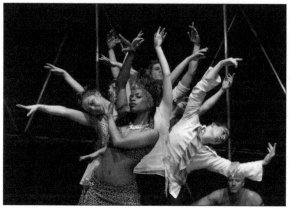

it's a big effort to blow-dry my hair so I'd rather just *not*, but I have to also understand the industry that I'm in and – not conform – but gently try and break the barriers. I don't want to put myself out of work, but I always find, once you've got your foot in the door, that's when you have to try and speak up. I find myself doing that now. I did two episodes on *Silent Witness* a few months ago and my character got her hair wet, and I said to them, "You know when my hair's wet it will be curly?" And they completely embraced it. They allowed me to wear more than one hairstyle throughout the duration of the filming. When my hair was wet they allowed me a day in between filming to get my hair back to the state it was in the beginning, and that was a really big thing for me, because normally I'm not allowed to change my hairstyle because it's not convenient. So to be in a show for only two episodes and be able to have hairstyles, I felt like Susan Kelechi Watson from *This is Us*, who has amazing hairstyles every episode, and then she wears her headscarves, and goes to bed with rollers in – I was like, that's perfect. So I felt a bit like her for a moment!

What do you think about how brands situate themselves in the narrative of Black hair? What more do you think could be done?

They're doing a brilliant job – it's come a long way in my lifetime. I'm very much into Shea Moisture at the moment because they cater to all hair types. I think I'm a 4B and my children range from 3A to 3C – we've all got different hair, but it's the one brand that we can all use. Usually, we're buying different things throughout the whole household which is quite costly and time consuming, and it clutters the bathroom, so with this we can all use something that's brilliant, organic and natural. More could be done in advertising. One of my friends did an advert for keratin but she didn't have keratin, and I know that's the case for Cheryl Cole who did an advert for L'Oréal but had extensions in. Let's have the naked truth – advertising doesn't need to be glossy, it just needs to be real, fun and vibrant. They need to be more honest with it, because people are going to try it and review it anyway, so if the reviews don't match the advert, you've lost. If advertising is honest, and the reviews are championing that, then the brands have won. So I think we need a bit more transparency, a bit more honesty and a bit more playfulness – you're trying to advertise things that people are going to factor into their lives. Our lives aren't meant to be serious – our lives are real, they're dynamic, so let art mirror life and life mirror art and all will be fine.

What do you think of the differences between the way Black men and Black women are treated in society when it comes to standards of beauty?

I find this question so brilliant and so difficult to answer, because I come from a family where I have one sister and one brother, and I've now got four boys. I think it's down to the individual, the industry, your audience and surroundings, and obviously what role you're playing. In the entertainment industry I still find that women are sexualized far too much, and I'm trying to educate my boys not to see them in that light. I think ultimately it comes down to us. If we want the narrative to change, we have to dictate the narrative – we have to speak up; if we see something wrong we have to call it out. I was offered a role a few years ago and I had to turn it down. It was for a great TV show but I said "No," because I didn't want to be the Black actor portraying that stereotypical character on film. They would never have asked a man to do it but they wanted a woman to do it, and I just thought, "No." I think in my industry especially, a lot of us say, "Yes" to the job. Understandably, you've got to pay the mortgage and raise your platforms and get out – but if you say "Yes" to that one wrong thing, it sets us all back 10 years because we all become the object of something.

What more do you think needs to be done to empower Black women, particularly regarding hair and beauty?

Smash all the rules. Because we talk about natural beauty, but if a woman walks in and she's wearing an Afro, you don't encourage her to get a perm or tell her to tie her hair back. If a woman wants to experiment with colour in her hair, just because it's in plaits doesn't mean you have to send her home, because if a Caucasian woman comes in with pink hair you're fine with it. It just takes one person to speak up or respectfully decline something for change to filter through.

What advice would you give to your younger self today? Or what do you wish your younger self had known, that you know today?

I'd tell her, "You are enough. You are unique, your uniqueness is beautiful, embrace it." I wish I had all of today's role models around when I was younger, but I'm grateful that I had my family because they played a big part in everything. I'm glad that things are changing and that we're moving forward.

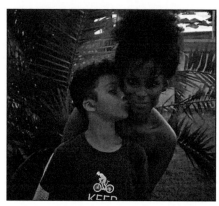

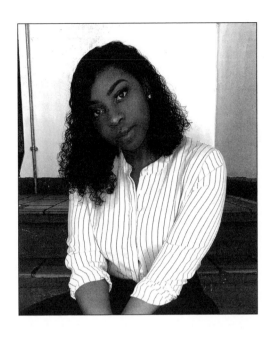

JAEL UMERAH-MAKELEMI

Jael Umerah-Makelemi is a London-based illustrator, art director and founder of Nubiart. Nubiart is an illustration studio that focuses on celebrating Black women, highlighting mental health and promoting self-care. She believes in empowerment through representation. She wants to inspire the next generation of creatives by showing them that they can do and create anything.

With her deep-rooted passion for fashion, many of her illustrations infuse African patterns with bright colour contrasts. Coming from a Nigerian background and living in South London, she has grown up in a diverse community. She has always been fascinated by the multitude of various and bold personalities who aren't afraid to express who they are through colour and fashion. This influenced her to create illustrations that are unapologetically vibrant and bold in style. Her art is primarily digital, but she has been exploring painting and sketching also.

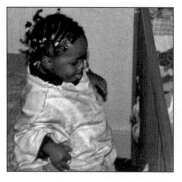

What was your go-to hairstyle as a child, and who used to do your hair?

My go-to hairstyle was single plaits – I absolutely loved them! It was a versatile hairstyle that allowed me to express myself. I'd try out different colours like burgundy, grey, purple, lilac etc. – the list goes on. My aunt was the only person who did my hair growing up because she was and still is the hair expert in the family.

Who was your hair inspiration growing up? Did you struggle to find Black hair inspiration?

My hair inspiration growing up was my aunt. I admired how long and healthy her natural hair was and aspired to get my hair to her level.

Outside of my family, I found it hard to find anyone who represented me on TV or in magazines. Everything was centred around Eurocentric features and beauty so I did go through a phase where all I wanted was my hair straightened and to try weave out. My mum actually didn't let me get my first weave until I was 16 going to prom. I didn't understand why then, but I'm thankful now as I have a whole new appreciation for my natural hair.

Who are the Black female role models in society, and how do they differ from the role models you had growing up?

My role model has always been my mum; the way she continues to elevate through adversity is inspirational. In terms of well-known women, I'm inspired by Rihanna, Michaela Coel, Dr. Shola Mos-Shogbamimu. They're all women who are strong not because they're Black or they're women, but because they're confident in who they are and aren't afraid to share their stories and opinions.

The role models available now are definitely different from the role models then. It was hard to find someone to look up to who you could relate to. We're still struggling with representing Black women across all industries to this day but it is a lot easier to find someone who looks like you.

When you were young, what beauty standards did you associate with being beautiful, and how do they differ today?

Everything was centred and still is centred around Eurocentric beauty standards. Most Black girls wanted straight hair – at one point I did too. I remember a period of time where I would constantly straighten my hair and ended up with heat damage; it took years for me to get my hair back to how it was. I don't think much has changed since then in terms of beauty standards, but I do see a lot more Black women embracing their natural hair.

At what age were you made to feel like your hair was different? Tell us about that experience, what it felt like and how you navigated that?

I always knew my hair was different, but I really understood how different it was in secondary school. I'd remember times when Black girls weren't allowed to wear brown extensions (even though some of our hair wasn't black), but students from European backgrounds were allowed to have highlights and amber. It didn't feel fair. Hair is the one way we can express ourselves, and to have that taken away did put a damper on my school experience.

What age were you when you started to make your own hair decisions, what were those decisions, and why did you choose the style you did?

I started to make my own hair decisions at 16, however I do remember a time when I decided to cut my own fringe (I was about 14 then). My mum and aunt loved fringes back then and I wanted to be like them. I remember going into school the next day feeling stunning, but by the end of the day my fringe had frizzed up and I vowed to never do DIY haircuts on myself again.

Do you have any experiences where your hair had a major effect on something in your life?

My hair definitely affected my confidence. When my hair was done in a way that I felt best expressed who I was, I felt untouchable. When it was in a hairstyle that I felt held me back (e.g. during secondary school), I regularly felt like there was nothing special about me.

How do you wear your hair at work? Or for interviews? Has this changed over time?

I don't really have a particular style that I wear to work. I do stick to dark brown most of the time, but I have gone to work with bright red amber and dark green hairstyles.

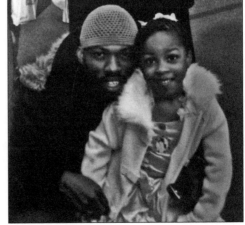

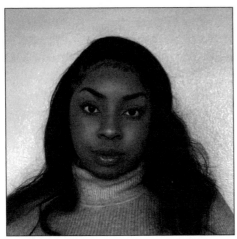

What part does your hair play in your life today? What in your "hair story" helped shape that?

My hair makes me feel beautiful. When I wear my natural hair, there's something in me that feels whole, like an elevated version of myself. Before the pandemic, I would go out with my hair up often as it made me feel like a new person. My hair has definitely become a way for me to feel confident.

What do you think about how brands situate themselves in the narrative of Black hair? What more do you think could be done?

More can be done to represent different hair types, such as products specifically for different hair textures. Everyone's hair is different and there's no "one product fits all" when it comes to haircare. I do want to see more Black-owned natural haircare brands as there are not enough in the mainstream limelight.

What do you think of beauty products such as skin-lightening creams?

There was a time when I did use a skin-lightening cream to try and lighten my knees when I was younger, but I very quickly realized that I need to learn to love my imperfections. Naturally, Black people have hyperpigmentation usually on their knees or armpits and that's something a lot of people try to get rid of till this day – but it's natural! I just want to encourage people to love the skin they're in, no matter what influences they see on social media or around them. Black is beautiful!

Can you easily find beauty products which suit your skin tone?

Now I can. I don't wear make-up often but when I do, I find it a lot easier to find my shade with brands like Fenty Beauty revolutionising the make-up industry. I've got yellow undertones and the foundation I used to use was either too yellow or orange, or made me look like a ghost. Thank you, Rihanna!

What do you think of the differences between the way Black men and Black women are treated in society when it comes to standards of beauty?

Both Black men and women have their own struggles and standards when it comes to beauty. I remember phases where it was all about lighter skin and being mixed race – if you didn't fit into that description then you weren't considered beautiful. Now we're seeing a celebration of darker tones, but there is still a long way to go when it comes to representing all types of Black people.

I do believe Black women have it harder. There's just a lot more for people to criticize. The things that we were taught were "ghetto" (braids, gelled baby hair, ponytails, long nails, etc.) are the same things that other ethnicities are being praised for. It does become difficult to just exist as a Black woman.

What more do you think needs to be done to empower Black women, particularly regarding hair and beauty?

Representation is key! Seeing more women at the top embracing their hair and beauty will definitely help. Additionally, a lot more needs to be done to combat the effect that social media has on people and their self-confidence. It's a really big factor in this conversation.

What advice would you give to your younger self today? Or, what do you wish your younger self had known, that you know today?

Embrace yourself, learn to love yourself and be unapologetic about who you are! Don't let anyone tell you how to wear your hair, experiment and wear what makes you feel like the queen you are. Also, hyperpigmentation is natural!

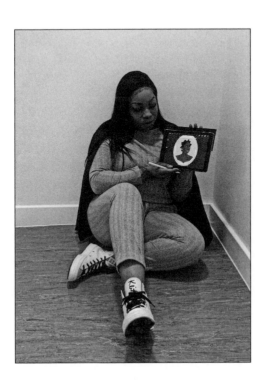

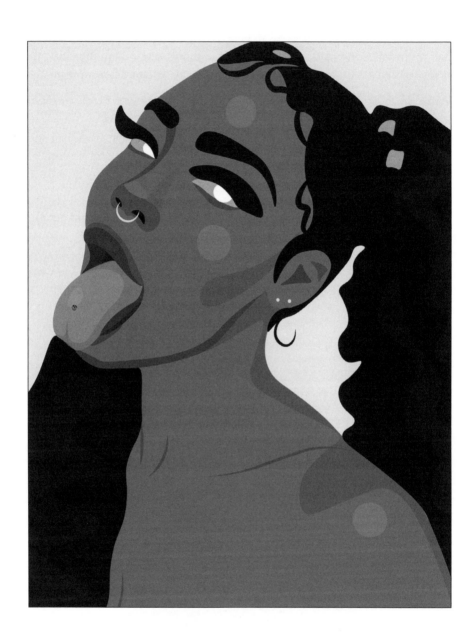

TOWEL TRESSES

My dream was
to wrap my hair in a towel,
twist it turban-like and after washing fling
it so that my long tresses wouldn't drip
down my back.

I put my hands in my hair,
tugged it to stretch it out,
still couldn't see it out of the corner of my
eye.
What kind of girl was I?

–Kadija Sesay

ENDNOTE

Saskia Calliste

We learn from the amazing women interviewed in this book that the practice of braiding, combing or plaiting our natural hair when we were children, which many of us endured rather than enjoyed, was an all-female ritual that taught many of us patience and strength.

African beauty was all that Black women knew before our ancestors were forcibly transported all over the world. We learn from our history that our hair was more than just a beauty choice. It was one of the ways that tribespeople in Africa could identify the tribe that a person belonged to simply by acknowledging their style. In the colonial era our hair helped us survive as Black slaves could feed themselves by concealing rice in their cornrows. In the 60s, wearing an Afro signified political and social resistance to discriminatory laws. Although those days are gone, how we choose to wear our hair when we roll out of bed in the morning still seems to mean more to others than it should.

The policing of Black hair is far from gone, and the pressures Black women face to conform have not been eliminated. These days, relaxing our hair is a non-desirable option for many of us, but it's clear from these pages that relaxing our hair was once considered a necessity if we wanted to fit into the beauty standards of Western society. The chemicals in relaxers have proved to be damaging, not only to our hair but to our health as well. Lye-based products have inextricable links to breast cancer, yet knowledge surrounding this devastating issue is fairly new. Companies which manufacture hair and beauty products have a responsibility to protect their customers from harmful chemicals but it seems that when it comes to Black women, this responsibility has long been either ignored or neglected. Most recently, Johnson & Johnson has been issued with a lawsuit by the National Council of Negro Women for targeting talcum-based products at Black women despite evidence that said products can cause ovarian cancer. As a Black woman, it's hard not to see these cases as the worst kind of exploitation of a community for financial gain.

However, what has changed now is our ability to connect with one another and find our community. Social media, education and shared experiences have allowed Black women to stand in solidarity with each other. When we cut through all the noise, we can recognize that we do and always have set the standards and trends others have tried to emulate. As the philosophy of diversity and inclusion changes hearts and minds, the dominance of Eurocentric beauty fades, and Black female beauty is shining through.

Today, in the same week, we can read one news headline about the Olympics banning Black swimmers from wearing swimming caps large enough to protect their hair, and then on a more positive note, we can read about how the British government has made it mandatory for trainee hairdressers in the UK to learn how to style and treat Black hair. Times are definitely changing, but like any social change, it seems like it's two steps forward, one step back.

Older generations of Black people marvel that Viola Davis, a dark-skinned woman, is leading a Hollywood TV show where she showcases a bonnet, braids, weave, twists – practically every common hairstyle known to Black women – remembering a time when the first African American Oscar-winner, Hattie McDaniel, had to sit at a segregated table at the back of the room at the 1940 Academy Awards Ceremony. Despite this snub, she made an impassioned speech, thanking the Academy for her Best Supporting Actress Award and their 'kindness.'

However, the ugly face of racism is still there. We saw it in the 2021 abuse and trolling of the English football team's Black players by those who refuse to accept that the diversity of people in our society is truly enriching. We see it with Meghan Markle and how the British press have treated her, making constant, unfair comparisons to the Duchess of Cambridge, Kate Middleton.

Reading "Her Hair Stories", it is interesting to note that no matter the difference in environment, family or social status, the interviewees share defining moments or experiences as part of their hair journeys – and sadly, many of them are negative. Participating in these interviews offered a form of catharsis for some who had not previously considered how much their hair journeys had shaped them. From having to cut off a lock of hair at someone's request, to not finding the right shade of make-up in a large store, these are experiences we minimize because they are a common occurrence, without realising the impact they have on how we see ourselves.

From Black influencers on social media to the rise in Black-owned businesses, Black creatives, Black artists, Black lawyers, Black MPs and Black scientists, we are forging successful careers, taking up space and making our voices heard. Whether it's Alicia Keys refusing to wear make-up on the red carpet or Jodie Turner-Smith playing Anne Boleyn, Black women are stepping forward into the spotlight and making choices for *themselves*.

This book and the stories it holds has not been created to sell you the myth that the struggle Black women face is over – because it's not.

Instead, it's a reminder that you can turn pain into something beautiful. To any Black girl or woman who has ever felt like less, this book is a reminder of your worth.

We hope that by reading about the energy and achievements of the incredible Black women in this book, you too will feel inspired to appreciate your natural beauty and to thrive in your own way. This is the Hairvolution, and it has only just begun.

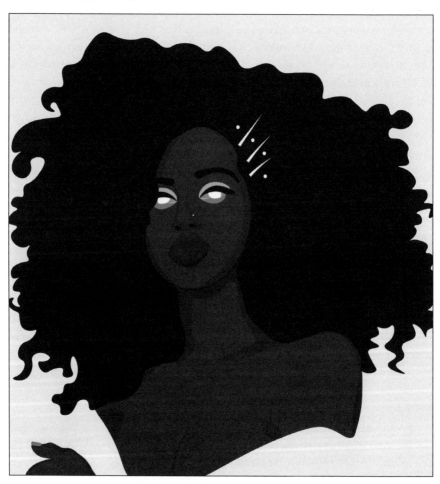

INDEX

INDEX